THE
SOPHROLOGY
METHOD

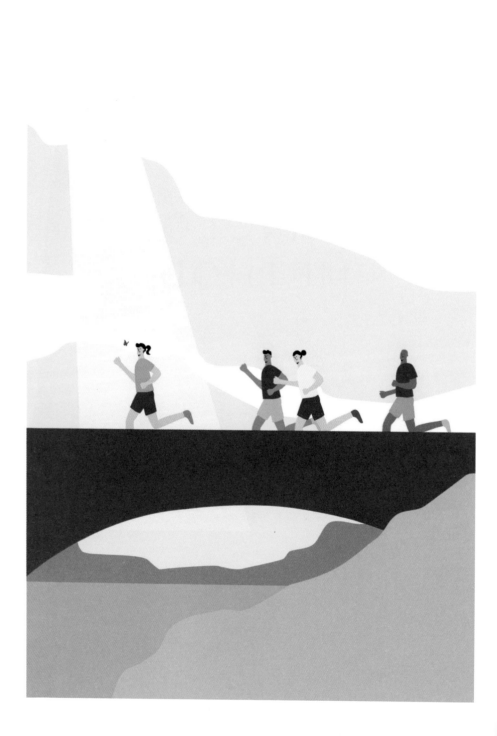

THE
SOPHROLOGY
METHOD

Simple mind–body
techniques for a
calmer, happier,
healthier you

FLORENCE PAROT

TO MY CHILDREN:
YOU HAVE TAUGHT ME EVERYTHING
I NEEDED TO KNOW.

An Hachette UK Company
www.hachette.co.uk

First published in Great Britain
in 2019 by Gaia, an imprint of
Octopus Publishing Group Ltd
Carmelite House
50 Victoria Embankment
London EC4Y 0DZ
www.octopusbooks.co.uk
www.octopusbooksusa.com

Text copyright © Florence Parot 2019
Design and layout copyright © Octopus
Publishing Group Ltd 2019

Distributed in the US by
Hachette Book Group
1290 Avenue of the Americas
4th and 5th Floors
New York, NY 10104

Distributed in Canada by
Canadian Manda Group
664 Annette St., Toronto,
Ontario, Canada M6S 2C8

ISBN: 978-1-85675-386-9

A CIP catalogue record for this book is available
from the British Library.

Printed and bound in China.

10 9 8 7 6 5 4 3 2 1

Commissioning Editor: Leanne Bryan
Art Director: Yasia Williams-Leedham
Assistant Editor: Nell Warner
Designer: Nicky Collings
Illustrator: Maia Boakye
Copy Editor: Caroline Taggart
Production Controller: Emily Noto

CONTENTS

INTRODUCTION

Sophrology is a mind–body method of healing and calming that is very new to some parts of the world but has been popular in France, Switzerland, Belgium and Spain for nearly 60 years. It is a modern technique that can be used for stress management, insomnia and anxiety; to prepare for public speaking or the stage or to enhance sports performance; in birth preparation, pain relief and much more.

The name Sophrology is based on the Greek words *sos* (harmony), *phren* (consciousness) and *logos* (study or science). Sophrology can therefore be described as the study of consciousness in harmony. It is a healthcare philosophy made up of very practical physical and mental exercises, in order to produce a clear and alert mind in a relaxed body.

As Michèle Freud, a famous French Sophrologist, puts it:

> "Sophrology helps to harmoniously develop our physical and psychological abilities and our inner resources, improve our performance, our imagination and creativity, focus and memorise. It improves sleep, helps overcome our fears and find our balance and joy in life. It uses imagination as a tool of change and evolution."

SOPHROLOGY CAN BE DESCRIBED AS THE STUDY OF CONSCIOUSNESS IN HARMONY.

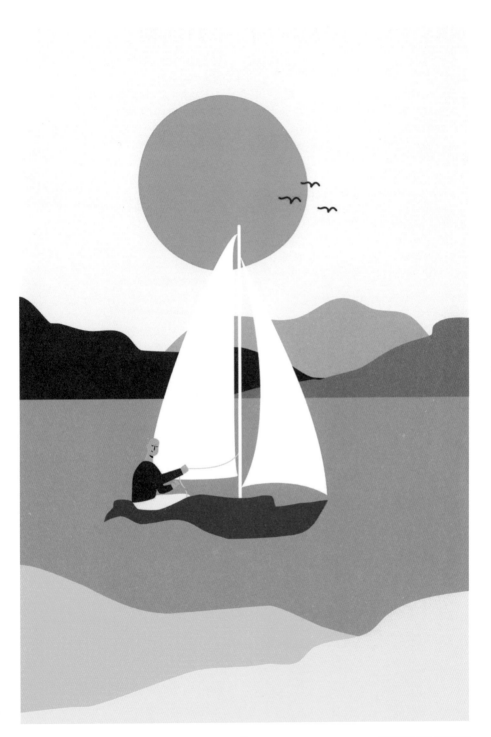

A BIT OF HISTORY

Sophrology was created in Spain in 1960 by a neuropsychiatrist called Professor Alfonso Caycedo (1932–2017). Professor Caycedo originally set out to find a way of healing depressed and traumatized clients by leading them to health and happiness with the lowest possible use of drugs and psychiatric treatments. He also wanted to study human consciousness and the means of altering its states and levels. He looked into clinical hypnosis, phenomenology and Western relaxation techniques as well as yoga, Buddhist meditation and Japanese Zen.

He approached each discipline, theory and philosophy with the intention of discovering what, exactly, improved people's health, both physically and mentally, in the fastest possible time and with lasting results. He studied in India, then travelled to Dharamsala to meet the Dalai Lama and study Buddhism. Lastly, he went to Japan to learn Zen in several monasteries. His idea was to help the Western mind use Eastern methods in a simple way, leaving aside philosophy and religion.

After returning to Spain, Professor Caycedo started to develop the concept of Sophrology. He initiated a Sophrology working group in Paris and spread the word at science conferences in Spain, Switzerland and Belgium.

In Switzerland, Dr Raymond Abrezol discovered the benefits of Sophrology and brought them to the attention of the general public. In 1965, he tried to help a friend with whom he played tennis regularly – the friend's performance and concentration improved dramatically. Abrezol then helped another friend with his skiing performance. Again, there was a dramatic improvement. In 1967, a Swiss ski coach, having heard about Dr Abrezol's work, asked him to help (in secret) train four skiers for the 1968 Grenoble Olympics. Three of them ended up on the Olympic podium. The athletes told the press about their Sophrology training and Abrezol found himself coaching the national skiing team from the next season. Medals started pouring in for Switzerland. Funnily enough, after the world championships in 1970, the Ski Federation asked Abrezol not to stay with the skiers at the starting point, arguing that he had too much influence on them and was "creating a disadvantage for other nations"! Abrezol went on to train many other athletes in a variety of sports, including sailing, boxing, cycling, tennis, water polo and golf. Between 1967 and 2004, Abrezol led skiers to win more than 200 Olympic medals.

Following this success, awareness of Sophrology grew rapidly throughout the French-speaking world. Although initially used only in medicine, its use soon spread into other areas. Sports, as we have seen, but also in the prevention of illness and promotion of health in the corporate world, as well as in education, the arts and other fields.

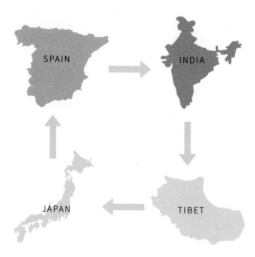

ALTHOUGH INITIALLY USED
ONLY IN MEDICINE, THE USE OF
SOPHROLOGY SOON SPREAD
INTO OTHER AREAS, NOT ONLY
IN SPORTS BUT ALSO IN THE
PREVENTION OF ILLNESS AND
PROMOTION OF HEALTH IN THE
CORPORATE WORLD, AS WELL
AS IN EDUCATION, THE ARTS
AND OTHER FIELDS.

WHAT CAN SOPHROLOGY DO?

In many European countries, Sophrology is used in a wide variety of settings. It is used in sports for self-confidence, motivation and team-building; to improve concentration, performance and energy levels, and cope with nerves and pressure… In the corporate world for stress and burnout management, repetitive strain injuries as well as body and mind tensions; to manage performance, energy levels and change; in preparation for interviews and public speaking; to improve self-confidence and control emotions; for self-development and improvement of interpersonal skills… In education for concentration, motivation and preparing for exams… Artists use it to boost creativity, for stage fright management and to improve memory and expression. It is also frequently used in a medical context to complement treatments for depression, phobias, addictions, anxiety and panic attacks; to prepare for an operation, manage pain, relieve insomnia and for prenatal and postnatal preparation. Generally speaking, you could say it is a balancing method, meant to help people feel better in their lives, giving them tools to enable them to grow and flourish, to be at their best when they most need to be.

WHO CAN BENEFIT?

Sophrology can help those dealing with stress, anxiety, low self-confidence, insomnia, burnout, chronic fatigue, pain and depression in the following areas:

- EVERYDAY LIFE -

- COMPETITIVE SPORTS -

- BUSINESS AND TEAM MANAGEMENT -

- STAGE PERFORMANCE -

- RELATIONSHIPS -

- EXAM PREPARATION -

- PUBLIC SPEAKING -

- INTERVIEWS -

SOPHROLOGY:
A CLEAR MIND IN A RELAXED BODY

Sophrology can be used just as well by the super-busy business person as by someone lying in a hospital bed. The whole idea is that it is simple and easy, anybody can do it and you don't need too much time on your hands. It fits into busy modern life. You learn exercises that you can then repeat on your own, that don't take long and that integrate easily into your day.

Sophrology is a structured set of exercises that can be done sitting down, standing up or even lying down if that is the only option for you (in cases of sickness or extreme fatigue, for instance). It is not a hands-on therapy. You close your eyes and follow simple instructions to learn how to relax, to experiment with different breathing techniques, to use simple movements and imagine situations or colours and so on.

In countries where Sophrology is well known, people tend to think of it as a relaxation technique. In reality, relaxation is just one of its many tools. If you are stressed or anxious, then relaxation could be what you are after. But if your goal is to be fully focused when speaking in public or to improve your performance when practising your favourite sports, what you need is the right amount of presence and energy and to be calm. Sophrology can help with this, too. Mainly, it makes us consciously, actively more aware of ourselves, how we feel and what we want. We take note of our environment. We work on our abilities and talents, a construction of the self in relation to others. We aim to be fully present and at our best whatever we are doing.

Sophrology is a very practical methodology, meant for everyday life. Although we start with focusing on ourselves and what is happening inside, it is not about shutting our eyes to what is going on in life. Quite the reverse. It is about becoming stronger and more aware so that we can be more alive and active in the world.

I WENT TO SEE FLORENCE FOR SOME SOPHROLOGY SESSIONS AND WAS AMAZED AT HOW EFFECTIVE THE TREATMENT WAS CONSIDERING IT IS SO GENTLE AND NON-INVASIVE.

CAROLINE RATNER

PRACTISING WITH FLORENCE PAROT SHOWED ME THE WAY TO KNOW MYSELF BETTER, MANAGE MY EMOTIONS, BECOME AWARE OF MY INNER RESOURCES AND STRENGTHS AND ENJOY BEING FULLY AND POSITIVELY ALIVE.

ISABELLE CASTELLANET

INTRODUCTION

THE SOPHROLOGY LEVELS

Sophrology is organized in 12 levels, although as a client, you will probably not be aware of this. The first four levels are those which are used more commonly in client practice.

LEVEL 1 is inspired particularly by yoga. It focuses on the body: how do I feel in my body, who am I inside? We become more aware of the body we are living in. We are focusing on living in the present, being present in our lives. We are introduced to relaxation in movement, body work, breath work and creative visualizations.

The goals are to get rid of our tensions, find inner harmony, improve our relationship with ourselves and develop our body awareness.

LEVEL 2 is inspired by Buddhist meditation. It focuses on the mind and on the five senses. We use contemplation as a tool: contemplating a simple object, contemplating ourselves as if from the outside (what am I?). We work on our future goals and projects, preparing for future events.

The notions we work on at this level that come directly from Buddhist meditation are: a peaceful mind, contemplation of an inner or external object, non-attachment.

The goals are to improve our relationship with others, developing our five senses and our intuition, enabling us to stand back, see things from a distance, let go.

LEVEL 3 is inspired by Japanese Zen. We focus on mind and body together as a whole. We use a meditative approach, learning to meditate in a simple, approachable way.

We become more aware of the world around us, meditating, trying to get to know the reality of things with a non-judgmental attitude and to experience the world as if we are seeing it for the first time.

We work on investigating the positive aspects of our past, in so far as it can help us live our present and future better, giving us the strength and ability to face them.

We experiment with sitting meditation (sitting on a chair, not in a lotus position) and walking meditation and awareness in every moment of everyday life.

In **LEVEL 4**, we return to the here and now, to being alive in the world in everyday life. We meditate to discover and conquer our existential or spiritual dimension. We also explore our life values, what gives meaning to our lives. Having progressed from Level 1, where we started exploring who we are and how we feel inside, we are now opening up to the world and discovering how to be truly ourselves in everyday life.

LEVELS 5 TO 8

At these levels, sound (the voice) is used to activate the body, mind and spirit. We focus on the awareness of vibrations in different parts of our body.

LEVELS 9 TO 12

In the last levels of Sophrology, we learn to live in full consciousness and to understand and be fully aware of the existential values of life: liberty, individuality. We continue to train to be fully present in each moment in time, but also to be aware of all the dimensions of space and time and to be fully in tune with ourselves, the world around us and the universe.

If this is beginning to sound complicated, remember that in Sophrology, what is really essential is that the technique helps you with everyday life. It is meant to be very practical, whether you are using it because you think it is fun (as it can be, for example if you use it as a tool to prepare for a stage performance), because you would like some help with a difficulty or as a general self-development tool.

THE PRINCIPLES OF SOPHROLOGY

OBJECTIVE REALITY AND NON-JUDGMENT

In Sophrology, what we call "objective reality" is a key concept. But what does it really mean?

Well, we are trying to have a non-judgmental attitude: looking at things as "neutrally" as possible, not using our previous knowledge or experience. We want to see the world with a child's mind, as if for the first time, listening to how we feel with no judgment or expectations.

We are learning to see things as much as possible as they really are, accepting the reality around us and accepting other people as they are, without ready-made ideas or assumptions. In Sophrology, whatever you are experiencing is OK – you are allowed to feel whatever you are feeling. Keeping an open mind, avoiding pre-judging and being present to whatever is around you starts in the Sophrology exercises and you then try to apply this to your everyday life.

POSITIVE ACTION

In Sophrology, we don't focus on the problem itself or on its causes. But we don't ignore it, either. Instead, to make ourselves better able to solve it, we put it aside for the duration of the session. We concentrate not on it but on the positive elements inside us and in our past, present or future that will enable us to move forward, to strengthen and reinforce the self, to reach our full potential. The assumption is that positive thoughts start a positive chain reaction inside us. According to Alfonso Caycedo, "Any positive action on the part of our consciousness affects our entire being." We ask ourselves: What makes me feel great? What brings me joy? Where do I take my energy from? And we use that knowledge.

Pascal Gautier, former Director of the Rennes School of Sophrology, put it this way:

> "Through an everyday practice, Sophrology aims at harmony in human beings: quite a feat! In practice, it does not mean seeing life through pink-tinted glasses, but putting an end to an unrealistic or negative vision of life to see things as they are (as much as possible) and reinforce whatever positive we have in us."

THE IMPORTANCE OF THE BODY

In Sophrology, we are exploring our inner self – body, mind and spirit. Sophrology gives us balance thanks to a gentler and better understanding of our own body, a calm and peaceful visit to it. First and foremost, the aim is to know ourselves better, to meet with our deeper selves, to be more at ease with ourselves, to accept ourselves the way we are.

It is about feeling more present, more aware of how we feel, fully alive here and now, and achieving harmony between body, mind and spirit. We want to get in touch with our body, improve our body perception, enjoy feeling alive.

FREEDOM, FLEXIBILITY

In Sophrology, we don't decide for others what suits them. You decide what is right for you and find your own way, taking into account how you feel and what is right for you in the moment.

For instance, if you are doing a standing exercise, you may wonder how to stand, how to place your body and your feet, whether you are doing the right thing and so on. In Sophrology there is no one answer to this. Of course, we could say that there is an anatomically correct way to stand. But correct for whom? We are all different. Sophrology gives us an answer that I find both simple and wonderful: stand as you like, in any way that feels comfortable to you today. What is appropriate for someone feeling fine may not be right for someone suffering from backache, or for the professional dancer whose lower body feels better with feet facing outward, or for someone in a wheelchair.

SOPHROLOGY GIVES US AN ANSWER
THAT I FIND BOTH SIMPLE AND
WONDERFUL: STAND AS YOU LIKE,
IN ANY WAY THAT FEELS COMFORTABLE
TO YOU TODAY.

FLORENCE PAROT

Sophrology is a structured method, but within that structure respecting how you feel is key. You learn to use the exercises by yourself, you make them yours, you own them. You are also free to feel whatever it is you are feeling.

Sophrology adapts to the person, the situation, the need, the context. There is no one way of doing things. If one technique does not work for you, there will be another that will. And if something is not possible for you, then adapt it.

Sophrology is a space of freedom. In this time and place, you are free to feel whatever it is you are feeling and to adapt the method to it.

As with life in general, it is about finding those moments when you are free to feel whatever you are feeling. You are free to decide how you will react to what someone tells you. In Sophrology, freedom to be yourself starts simply with the freedom to place your feet exactly how you like!

WHAT HAPPENS IN A SOPHROLOGY SESSION?

If at some point you have the opportunity or the interest to try a session with a Sophrologist, what can you expect? Well, you can have a one-to-one session or be part of a group. Although a group session may have a particular theme or setting, the goal is usually general wellbeing, mild stress management and life balance. A one-to-one session is likely to focus on a specific difficulty you are facing, with the Sophrologist guiding you through exercises that are tailor-made for you.

A one-to-one series of sessions always starts with a consultation in which the Sophrologist looks at what takes you there and whether or not Sophrology is likely to be able to help you. Each session will then have specific exercises you will work on and tools that you will learn to use on your own. Each session ends with discussing how the exercises went, how you felt and how to use the exercises in everyday life, how to practise.

Typical Sophrology practices include:

DYNAMIC RELAXATION

Sets of simple, gentle movements that are performed standing or sitting, normally with eyes closed, while you focus on your body and how you feel. The movements are usually easy – it is not about physical performance, more about presence and concentration on the body, rediscovering it. Most people think about their body mainly when it hurts. If you don't agree, let me ask you this: when was the last time you thought about your right big toe? See what I mean? In Sophrology we are what we call "present in the body" – we are very aware of the body and of its movement, because movement helps with focus and also because movement helps with such things as releasing tension.

The Shoulder Pumping exercise (see page 88) is a good example: in it you simply move your shoulders up and down, but as you synchronize your breath with the movement you need to focus. As you gently shake your shoulders, you release potential tensions there and become more aware of that part of your body.

BREATH AWARENESS

Nothing complex here: this usually starts with noticing how you breathe. Then, depending on your ability and how much practice you have already done, you may be given specific exercises. These will be simple, gentle techniques, so don't worry if you think you are not very adept at that sort of thing: it is about what you can do, not what anyone else thinks you should be doing! Again, it is more important to notice, to become more aware of your body and how you feel, than to execute perfect breathwork. All the exercises are adapted to your abilities and how you feel in the moment. For instance, how are you breathing right now? See, you have started working with your breath!

VISUALIZATION

When we talk about visualization in Sophrology, we mean "imagining" rather than "seeing", so if you have no idea where to start with visual imagery, don't panic: again, it is about going with what you can do and taking it from there, perhaps using other senses – hearing, touch – to help you imagine… Suggestion is left to a minimum to let each person practise the exercise in their own way. Take the example of imagining yourself in a safe, peaceful landscape – a classic visualization technique. When we use this in Sophrology, the idea is not to give you a detailed version of what your landscape "should" be like. We prefer to let you look for your own, searching inside yourself to see what really excites you and working with that. A client of

mine once ended up imagining he was paragliding. He loved it and found it very empowering. It was definitely not something I would have suggested, as I am afraid of heights!

The mind–body connection is essential in Sophrology. As you will see, we work with both in the different types of exercises we use. So you could say we have "mind" exercises (such as visualization) and "body" exercises (such as gentle movements) as well as "mind–body" exercises (such as walking meditation). This is not just to provide a variety of exercises so that you can choose what works best for you. It is above all because Sophrology considers the human being as a whole: body, mind, emotions, spirit, all together as one, functioning together and therefore needing to be looked at as one.

A TYPICAL SESSION

Most Sophrology is done with the eyes closed. It nearly always starts with what we call a body scan (see page 20) or at least a focusing exercise. The body scan is important in that it prepares you for the rest of the practice, giving you time to settle down, to calm yourself, to direct your focus inside you, concentrating on what you feel and what is happening in your mind and body, so that you forget about what is happening in your life for a little while. Your attention shifts and your level of awareness changes. You are more in tune with your inner life, more focused.

Now you move on to the practice itself, which is either dynamic relaxation, breathing awareness, visualization or a combination of the three. You always take time to listen to how you are feeling at the end of the practice and usually in between each exercise within the practice. The aim is not necessarily to feel "good" or relaxed. Whatever you are feeling is right – there is no "should" or "must".

You first notice how you feel, then you can decide what you do with it. The most important thing is to reconnect to your body, your thoughts, your sensations and emotions, even if only for a moment, during the exercise. You learn or rediscover what it is to listen in, to truly feel, with no expectations, no judgment, no filters from the outside world. You end with taking time to come back to the room and your usual level of awareness (see page 20). You then take some time to write about the whole experience or to share it out loud if you are practising with others.

WHATEVER YOU ARE FEELING IS RIGHT – THERE IS NO "SHOULD" OR "MUST".

So, to recap, the classic format of a Sophrology exercise is:

- BODY SCAN -

- PRACTICE
(DYNAMIC RELAXATION,
BREATH AWARENESS,
VISUALIZATION, AND SO ON) -

- LISTENING TO HOW YOU
ARE FEELING -

- COMING BACK TO THE ROOM -

- REFLECTING ON THE
EXPERIENCE-

Now let's look at two of those aspects in more detail.

THE BODY SCAN

Typically, during a body scan, you concentrate on your body from head to toe, bit by bit, slowly or quickly. This could take anything from two to ten minutes, depending on how experienced you are or what is relevant for today, how much time you have, how you feel and so on. So a basic body scan could look something like this:

- Sit down or stand in a comfortable position and close your eyes. Take a few moments to feel your body as a whole from head to toe, especially the places where you are in contact with the floor or with your chair, simply the way your body is placed.

- Focus on your head and face. Be very present there. Sense how you feel and try to imagine calmness and relaxation settling in. Unclench your jaw. Imagine your brain resting, your mind becoming quiet. If ideas come and go, let them simply flow past or imagine you are putting them in a bag outside the door – you can deal with them later. If your mind wanders off at any point, bring it back, gently reminding it to focus on what you are doing.

- Now move your attention down to your throat and neck. Imagine more space inside as if to let more air through. Imagine your neck muscles unknotting.

- Relax your shoulders, letting them drop gently toward the floor. Focus on your upper arms, your elbows, forearms, wrists and hands, right to the tips of your fingers.

- Now bring your awareness to your chest and upper back, breathing gently.

- Focus on your abdomen and lower back. Imagine all the organs inside working together in harmony.

- Move your attention down to the lower part of your body, your hips and legs. Sense how your legs are placed, focus on your feet down to the soles, your toes.

- You are aware of your whole body from head to toe.

COMING BACK TO THE ROOM

At the end of the practice, bring yourself slowly "back to the room". Become gradually more aware of the environment, of where you are, of all the elements surrounding you: the furniture, the temperature of the room, noises... Gently start moving your toes, legs, fingers, arms; move your shoulders, neck, head... gently stretch, rub your hands and yawn if you want to. When you are ready, open your eyes. This is an important part of the practice, ensuring that you come back to your usual level of alertness, rather than feeling drowsy.

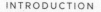

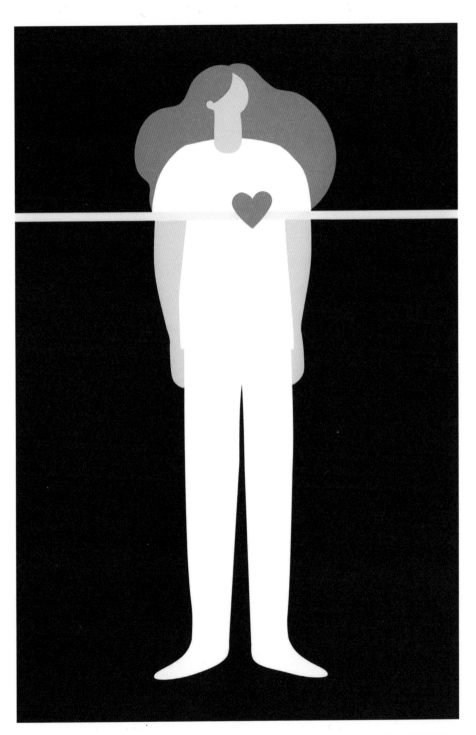

HOW TO GET STARTED

One of the great attractions of Sophrology is how easy it is to get started. You don't need any particular equipment or specific clothes. You don't need to go to a gym or anywhere else special. The idea is that Sophrology adapts to your life, not the other way round. So you can practise "as you are", in any clothes at all, whether they are something comfortable at home or a suit and tie or high heels at work.

You don't need to have particular circumstances, either. Of course, it may be inappropriate (or downright dangerous) to practise dynamic relaxation in the middle of the street, but there are some exercises you can do anywhere, even in a full meeting room. And you can always find a quiet corner to do something a bit more noticeable. This means no special candles, lighting or cushions and no music. Of course, if that's what you like when you are at home, go ahead and use them. But the general idea is that you are learning skills you want to be able to use anywhere, not just when you are in the right environment.

In other words, for Sophrology, you only need yourself as you are, and a simple upright chair for some of the exercises.

> THE IDEA IS THAT SOPHROLOGY ADAPTS TO YOUR LIFE, NOT THE OTHER WAY ROUND.

POSTURES

Most Sophrology exercises are performed either standing up or sitting on an ordinary, upright chair. But again, you adapt to your circumstances: where you are and what you can do on that particular day. If you can't stand or are too tired even to sit up, you can lie down. Always do whatever feels most comfortable for you. So although throughout the book I will suggest the most common posture for each exercise, remember that you can always adapt to what works best for you.

Do the exercises at your own pace – be very gentle with yourself and do what feels possible. Sophrology offers a variety of different tools, so start with what feels right – the idea is to try different ways and see what works for you.

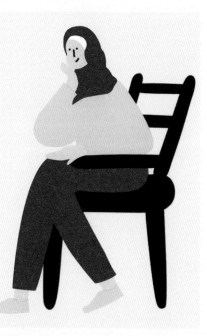

BREATHING

In Sophrology, we always breathe in through the nose. You can then breathe out either through the nose or through the mouth, depending on the exercise and on what feels right for you.

You will notice I don't recommend any particular type of breathing in this book. You don't have to breathe from your chest, your abdomen or your diaphragm (the large flat muscle under the lungs). This is because in Sophrology the most important aspect of breathing is becoming aware of *how* you are breathing at the moment, not necessarily changing it and definitely not checking whether you are doing it "right" or "wrong". This is simply because we use breathing first and foremost as a tool to make us more aware of our body, and because we don't want to force anything. The more you learn to pay attention to your breathing, to stop and pause, the more your breathing will slow down and expand naturally. So you could say we are looking ultimately for a gentle, deep, slow breath – a full breath, as some would call it. But it's important to let it fall into place naturally. So, if you follow what I suggest for each exercise but adapt it to what feels most natural to you, without forcing anything, you will be on the right Sophrological track.

THE MORE YOU LEARN TO PAY ATTENTION TO YOUR BREATHING, TO STOP AND PAUSE, THE MORE YOUR BREATHING WILL SLOW DOWN AND EXPAND NATURALLY.

TIMING AND REPETITION

You can practise the exercises in this book as often and for as long as you like. For instance, you may want to do at least a few minutes a day or maybe a longer exercise once a week. But whatever you choose, repetition is key and the exercises will have more impact if you practise them often. I have given guidelines on page 28 on preparing your own Sophrology programme and for each exercise as they appear in the subsequent chapters, I have included an idea of how long it may take (what I call "standard timing"), but this is just for guidance: feel free to adapt to your situation or simply to the time you have to hand.

SOPHROLOGY DRASTICALLY TRANSFORMED MY LIFE FROM ONE OF OVERWHELMING STRESS TO ONE OF HARMONY.

ISABELLE CASTELLANET

HOW TO USE THIS BOOK

This book is meant as an introduction to the Sophrology method and as a practical guide to help you get started on many of the issues Sophrology can help with.

In each chapter, you will find:

PRACTICAL TIPS

that are short guidelines for everyday use, to try here and there when you want.

QUICK EVERYDAY TOOLS

that you can start implementing in your life straight away. Some of them take longer than the shorter practise-at-home techniques – the longest require perhaps 15 minutes – but the point about these tools is that they can easily be used anywhere and at any time.

PRACTISE-AT-HOME TECHNIQUES

for which you will need to set aside some time, from as little as five minutes, never more than thirty. For these you will need to make sure you have peace and quiet.

Always go with what feels easiest and simplest when following what is suggested here. I repeat: there is no one way to do things in Sophrology. It is important that you notice how you feel and what you can do and take it from there. If standing is uncomfortable, for instance, it is OK to sit down. You know best. Adapt to what works for you.

There are two ways to use this book: practise and try the tips and tools whenever you feel like it, or put together some form of training practice for yourself. Whether or not you work in a structured way, remember that the more you repeat the exercises the more effective they will be. I suggest possible training programmes on page 28 but they are examples and you can definitely create your own, depending on what you want to focus on. Please note that it is worth starting your Sophrology practice when all is well, rather than waiting until you reach a crisis in your life: that way you can find the tool you can use when you need it most.

A WORD ABOUT
HEALTH CONCERNS

Remember that this book is meant as a general introduction to Sophrology, to give you an idea of what it is about and maybe even encourage you to implement some changes in your life, but, especially if you are facing a particular difficulty, I would recommend consulting a Sophrologist in person who will be able to listen to your needs, assess the situation and guide you in more depth. They will also know how to put together a tailor-made plan for you.

Sophrology sessions traditionally happen face-to-face but, with the development of modern technologies, it has now become possible to have them using Skype. A "live" face-to-face session is a great experience but if you do not have a Sophrologist near you geographically, this is definitely an alternative worth exploring. Check the list of resources on page 205 to help you find a practitioner who offers this service.

Of course, if you have any concerns about your health, are not sure what to do or are worried about particular sensations or symptoms, do consult a doctor for medical advice. Sophrology in general and this book in particular are not intended to diagnose medical conditions or replace your healthcare professional.

PRACTISING SOPHROLOGY

Before we start a practice, we take time to become aware of our body, to focus on it bit by bit – checking in, as it were (see the Body Scan, page 20). If we notice tension, we may try to relax it, but never force anything, nor try too hard. Depending on what you are working on, the awareness itself may be the main focus. Or it may be the relaxation. Or both. In most of the exercises in this book, whether "quick everyday tools" or "practise-at-home techniques", I recommend some form of body scan as an introduction. But it can be very short, a few minutes. Or longer if this is what you need. For the "quick everyday tools", you can also jump into them without a body scan if you need something super-quick in an emergency.

At the end of each practice, take a couple of minutes to listen to how you feel before stretching and opening your eyes.

Immediately after that, in a typical Sophrology session, you would take time to give some feedback on the practice. If you were working with a Sophrologist, you would tell them how you felt and how the exercise went. On your own, it is a great idea to keep a journal about it, so if you want to write in a notebook after every practice, do so.

> AFTER A FEW MONTHS OF REGULAR PRACTICE OF SOPHROLOGY, I FEEL ABLE TO RELAX AND CONCENTRATE WHENEVER I NEED TO.
>
> CHRISTINE PIGNET

YOUR SOPHROLOGY JOURNAL

Use your Sophrology journal to record how you felt during each session. Was your body tingling, heavy, tired…? What about your mind? Was it focused or distracted? Peaceful or still anxious? Did you have any bright ideas or make any great discoveries? Instead, you could use the notes page at the end of each chapter.

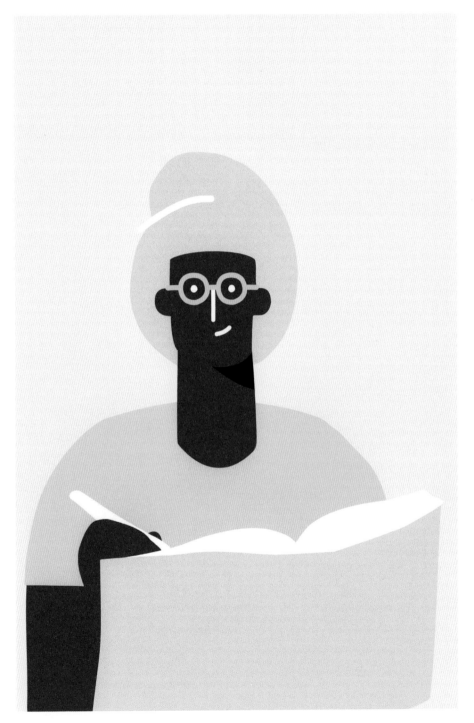

INTRODUCTION

PUTTING TOGETHER A SOPHROLOGY PROGRAMME

Choose a couple of "everyday tools" in the book and practise them every day at the time of your choice for a week. It may be easier to practise at the same time every day in order to get into the habit, but you can practise Sophrology at any time. Change exercises every week. Over time you may find yourself using a bunch of your favourites every day and others for specific circumstances.

Once a week, when you have more time, go through a longer "practise-at-home" technique. Take your time, write your feedback in your journal. Enjoy this time for yourself!

If you are more interested in a particular topic, such as preparing for an exam or improving your sporting performance, start with the exercises in the relevant chapter and practise them often. As you progress, add in a few more from other chapters (I give you suggestions at the end of each chapter for exercises that will complement what you are doing).

Remember that practising at least once a day, even for a few minutes, is more efficient than doing the exercises sporadically.

As with other forms of exercise and healing, however much fun it is to discover a technique through a book, nothing much will improve if you don't practise. In Sophrology, repetition is key.

> REMEMBER THAT PRACTISING AT LEAST ONCE A DAY, EVEN FOR A FEW MINUTES, IS MORE EFFICIENT THAN DOING THE EXERCISES SPORADICALLY.

THE SOPHROLOGY METHOD AUDIO

You can access audio versions of the following Sophrology exercises from this book at http://florence-parot.co.uk

SOME SAMPLE PROGRAMMES

To help you get started, here are a few examples that you might try for the first couple of weeks. These are just suggestions, to give you ideas – feel free to do what feels right for you!

EXAMPLE 1

Week 1
Every day: Neck Exercise (see page 54) and Shoulder Pumping (see page 88); once a week: Landscape Visualization (see page 164)

Week 2
Every day: The Target (see page 68) and Tense and Release (see page 89); twice a week: Breathe in the Sunshine (see page 139) and Five Senses (see page 119)

EXAMPLE 2

Week 1
Every day: The Puppet (see page 36), Forearms Exercise (see page 38) and Walking on the Spot (see page 39); once a week: Coloured Nature Visualization (see page 40)

Week 2
Every day: Grounding: Rooted Like a Tree (see page 121) or Grounding: Beam of Light (see page 136) and Shoulder Pumping (see page 88); once a week: Energy Pyramid Visualization (see page 41)

EXAMPLE 3

Week 1
Every morning: Neck Exercise (see page 54), Shoulder Pumping (see page 88) and The Puppet (see page 36); before going to bed: Relaxing Counted Breathing (see page 106) and Tense and Release (see page 89)

Week 2
Every morning: Breathe in the Sunshine (see page 139) and Five Senses (see page 119); before going to bed: Relaxing Counted Breathing (see page 106) and Tense and Release (see page 89)

INTRODUCTION

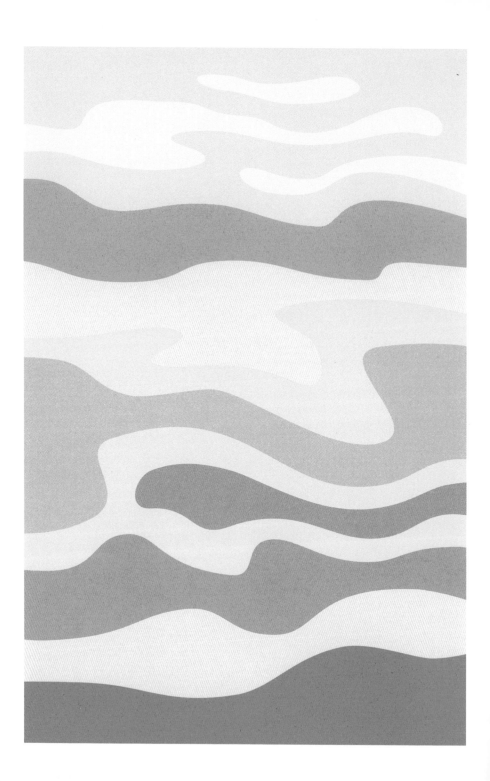

1
IMPROVE ENERGY LEVELS

USING SOPHROLOGY
TO BOOST YOUR ENERGY

As I have said, relaxation techniques are a part of Sophrology, but only a part. Sophrology is first and foremost about balance, so sometimes we do need relaxation, but sometimes we need more energy.

Think about getting ready to run a marathon. You may need some level of relaxation if you are feeling anxious about it but you will mainly need plenty of energy, focus, presence. Sophrology will not replace training for the race, sleeping well and eating properly, but it will be a worthwhile complement to all this in order for you to be at your best when you most need to be.

> SOPHROLOGY WILL NOT REPLACE TRAINING FOR THE RACE, SLEEPING WELL AND EATING PROPERLY, BUT IT WILL BE A WORTHWHILE COMPLEMENT TO ALL THIS IN ORDER FOR YOU TO BE AT YOUR BEST WHEN YOU MOST NEED TO BE.

The first level of Sophrology focuses on the body, on being more present, more aware of how you feel. The aim is to know yourself better, first to accept yourself the way you are and whatever you are feeling. Then to empower you to decide what to do with this knowledge. For instance, if what you are feeling right now is tired, you may not listen to your body and be in denial of this fatigue, thinking, "I am fine, thank you very much." Not acknowledging your tiredness could lead to complete exhaustion, burnout or illness. But acknowledging right now that what you are feeling is tired and that maybe there is a good reason for it (allowing yourself to truly feel this – yes, you are entitled to feel tired!) is good in itself. You can then decide what you will do about it: are you going to power through because you have so much work and tomorrow is a weekend anyway; take a break for a few minutes; or take the day off? The choice is yours, but it is at least a more enlightened one. Accepting what you are feeling could therefore help prevent bad decisions. For instance, going back to that marathon, if you decide to run but are exhausted, you could end up injuring yourself, whereas if you had paid attention to that twinge in your ankle earlier on, that injury might not have happened. Being fully present in the body will also mean that when you feel amazing, you will feel it even more!

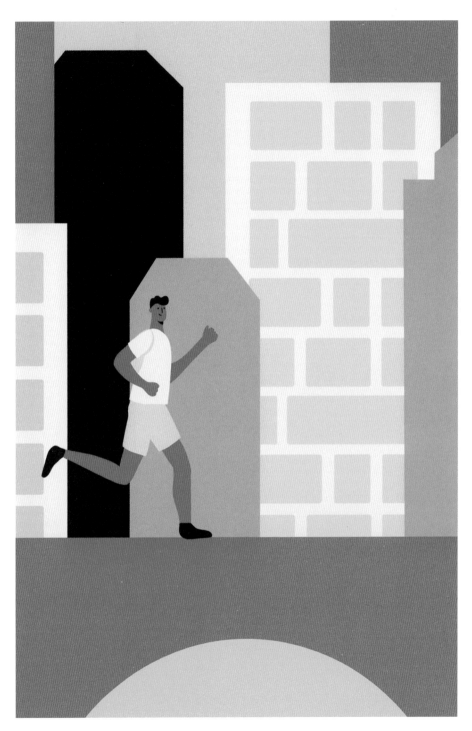

IMPROVE ENERGY LEVELS

BODY AWARENESS IS KEY

So what does all this have to do with your energy levels? Well, as with everything in Sophrology, it starts here with body awareness. Be present in the body and to the body, take good care of it (not just superficially), live in harmony with it and already your energy levels will feel very different. Because if you listen to your body, you will know to stop before you become exhausted; you will know when to refuel or sleep, and what best to eat or drink. As well as this, Sophrology also has a number of exercises that you can use when you need to feel the power even more, practices which use the force of the imagination to bring in more energy or to go for that one movement that will stimulate the whole body.

So this is what you are going to do here: be present to the body and in the body. And have a look at a few techniques to give you an extra boost when you need it.

> BE PRESENT IN THE BODY AND TO THE BODY, TAKE GOOD CARE OF IT, LIVE IN HARMONY WITH IT AND ALREADY YOUR ENERGY LEVELS WILL FEEL VERY DIFFERENT.

PRACTICAL TIPS

TAKE A BREAK

I will repeat this a number of times in the course of the book: take a break *before* you are tired. You will restore your energy more quickly and be effective and feel alert much longer. Take regular short breaks throughout the day (see page 150 for more on this).

A QUICK AND EASY "ON THE SPOT" CHECK

Close your eyes right now in the position you are in and, without changing anything, check how you are feeling. Do you feel relaxed? Stressed out? Don't judge, simply observe. Do you need to change something in order to feel better? Go ahead. Now, how does that feel? Good? Enjoy it. And then open your eyes, of course!

BREATHING AWARENESS

Sit down and notice how you are breathing. Don't change anything. Just follow the rhythm of your breath: its pattern, its speed, how it feels. Maybe you can notice the air coming in and out when you breathe, the path it is following inside you. And what about the places in your body that move when you breathe? Maybe your shoulders, maybe your chest, maybe your abdomen. This is not about telling you how to breathe, there is no "right" or "wrong", no judgment involved. It is about discovering, noticing, being more able to feel what is happening in your body.

QUICK EVERYDAY TOOLS

THE PUPPET

Standard timing: 5 minutes

In this dynamic relaxation exercise, you jump up and down gently like a puppet with no strings. It is a very free, usually energizing movement. Don't do this if you have any problems with your knees or back. If you can't jump safely, try just bobbing up and down jelly-like with your feet firmly on the floor. Or move on to another exercise in this section.

1. Standing up and with your eyes closed, perform the body scan described on page 20.

2. Jump gently up and down while letting your body follow the movement in a very soft and relaxed way. Breathe naturally. Stop when you feel you have done enough.

3. Take a little time to listen to how you are feeling.

4. Come back into the room as described on page 20.

How do you feel?

Feel free to record your observations in your Sophrology journal or on the notes page at the end of this chapter.

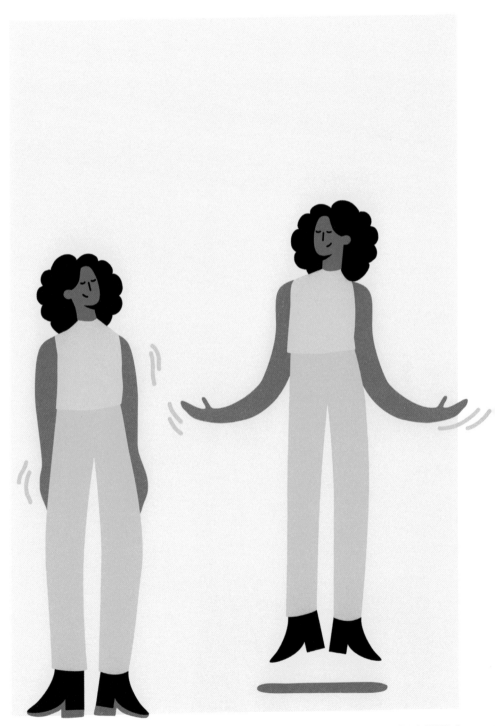

IMPROVE ENERGY LEVELS

FOREARMS EXERCISE

Standard timing: 5 minutes

You can easily do this gentle dynamic relaxation exercise sitting down if standing is difficult for you. Use it purely for body awareness or use your imagination for a specific intention, such as breathing in energy with each breath.

1. Standing up and with your eyes closed, perform the body scan described on page 20.

2. Keep the upper portion of your arms by your sides and just lift your forearms. Breathing in, let your hands go to your shoulders; breathing out, let them go back down, synchronizing the movement with your breathing. Do this for the length of time that feels right for you. You can simply focus on the movement and the breathing or you can imagine that each time you breathe out you are letting go of stress, tensions... and each time you breathe in you are bringing in peace, energy, calmness... whatever you need.

3. Come back into the room as described on page 20.

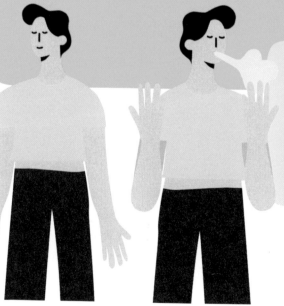

How do you feel?

Feel free to record your observations in your Sophrology journal or on the notes page at the end of this chapter.

WALKING ON THE SPOT

Standard timing: 5 minutes

This dynamic relaxation exercise mimics walking while staying where you are. You can play with different speeds. It is about noticing the differences in your body, noticing the movement itself, starting to put energy in motion and preparing for the next step in your day.

1. Standing up and with your eyes closed, perform the body scan described on page 20.

2. Slowly and gently start walking on the spot, noticing the movements of your feet and legs, the points of contact with the floor. Your arms do not move, they are just gently present at each side. Increase the speed for a short while and then slow down again. Simply notice how you feel.

3. Come back into the room as described on page 20.

How do you feel?

Feel free to record your observations in your Sophrology journal or on the notes page at the end of this chapter.

PRACTISE-AT-HOME TECHNIQUES

COLOURED NATURE VISUALIZATION

Standard timing: 15–20 minutes

This exercise suggests visualizing different aspects of a landscape with an emphasis on colours. It is more guided than most Sophrology visualizations, but feel free to find your own images to go with the colours or even imagine bathing in the colours themselves or breathing them in.

1. Sitting down and with your eyes closed, perform the body scan described on page 20.

2. Imagine yourself in front of a huge field of poppies. A red sun is rising on the horizon. You are bathing in this light, intense and positive. You breathe it in and let it spread inside you. You are becoming this red colour. You absorb all its energies.

3. Imagine walking past a beautiful orange grove. Its colour spreads into the air and into your body. You breathe it in and let it spread inside you.

4. The sun is now high in the sky and you are bathing in its golden yellow light while walking in a sunflower field. You breathe the colour in and let it spread inside you. You absorb all its energies.

5. You have reached a very green meadow, at the heart of a huge forest. Here, too, you let yourself be immersed in the colour, imagining a green blanket enveloping you.

6. Following your path, you get to the sea, of a deep blue, like the sky above you. You bathe in that deep, rich blue colour.

7. Night has come and the stars are above you in an indigo sky. You are in harmony with the sky and stars.

8. At dawn, the day breaks again and the sun shines on lilac flowers…

9. Imagine you are breathing in the energy of all these colours at once.

10. Then let go of all the images and listen to how you are feeling here and now.

11. Come back into the room as described on page 20.

How do you feel? Was visualizing easy or did you prefer just focusing on the colour or even your breath? This could be an interesting indication of which type of exercise works better for you.

Feel free to record your observations in your Sophrology journal or on the notes page at the end of this chapter.

ENERGY PYRAMID VISUALIZATION

Standard timing: 10–15 minutes

This exercise is about imagining you are bringing energy to the whole body.

1. Sitting down and with your eyes closed, perform the body scan described on page 20.

2. You are walking in a forest, a beautiful, colourful, tropical forest with tall trees. Take time to look around and enjoy the place. Then you arrive at a clearing and see a huge crystal pyramid in the middle, glittering in the sun.

3. You go in and find yourself in amazing sunlight. It is vibrating through the pyramid.

4. Lie down in the centre, right under the highest point of the pyramid.

Beams of golden energy are coming toward you, shining on you and giving you a bright energy that circulates in your whole body. Imagine a very fine golden beam shining on your forehead, on your stomach or anywhere on your body that feels right. Breathe in this energy and let it flow everywhere in your body. Remain there for as long as you feel necessary.

5. Go out of the pyramid, take your time, breathe. Then let go of the images you have created.

6. Listen to how you are feeling.

7. Come back into the room as described on page 20.

How do you feel? Did you use the sunbeam on a particular part of your body? Were there any specific sensations in that part of your body? Take time to really be at one with those sensations.

Feel free to record your observations in your Sophrology journal or on the notes page at the end of this chapter.

OTHER TECHNIQUES
TO COMPLEMENT THIS

**ALL DYNAMIC
RELAXATION EXERCISES**
(SEE PAGES 54, 55, 68, 72, 88,
89, 108, 121, 136, 160, 180, 182,
197, 198)

**FIVE SENSES
PRACTICAL TIP**
(SEE PAGE 119)

**BREATHE IN
THE SUNSHINE**
(SEE PAGE 139)

YOUR NOTES

IMPROVE ENERGY LEVELS

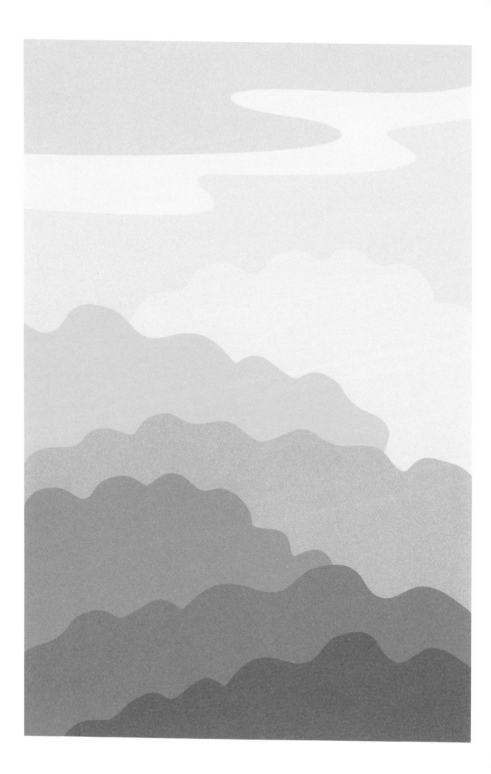

2
FOCUS THE MIND

USING SOPHROLOGY TO FOCUS

The second level of Sophrology focuses on the mind. It is not about emptying it or trying to think about nothing, but rather about focusing on something with the mind: you'll find that it is easier to think about something than think about nothing! You should preferably focus on something positive, such as following your breathing, or on an object (see the Neutral Object visualization on page 58). It could also be about being fully aware of a movement.

The idea is to focus the mind on one thing and one thing only, to reduce the amount of "stuff" going on in your head, stop the incessant chatter and use your mind to its full capacity.

> **THE IDEA IS TO FOCUS THE MIND ON ONE THING AND ONE THING ONLY, TO REDUCE THE AMOUNT OF "STUFF" GOING ON IN YOUR HEAD, STOP THE INCESSANT CHATTER AND USE YOUR MIND TO ITS FULL CAPACITY.**

BEING IN THE MOMENT VERSUS MULTITASKING

Did you know that our ability to focus has dramatically decreased over recent decades? Our attention is more and more fragmented. Nicholas Carr, in his book *The Shallows*, talks about a web-induced attention-deficit society. The increasing use of screens in the form of TV, phones, computers and other devices is one of the main reasons. They cause dispersion and distraction. Before you start arguing about this, take note of how many times you check a screen in the next couple of hours and how often you switch from one thing to another. Really notice… see what I mean? This is not a very efficient way to function: some studies show that if we are interrupted, we can take up to 25 minutes to regain the same amount of focus. Others suggest that if we have a screen near us, we cannot truly focus for more than three minutes at a time. Three minutes… How do you expect to do what you have to do properly? Imagine the quality of your work if your flow is broken every three minutes! And we have not even talked about other interruptions: people walking into your office, the phone ringing…

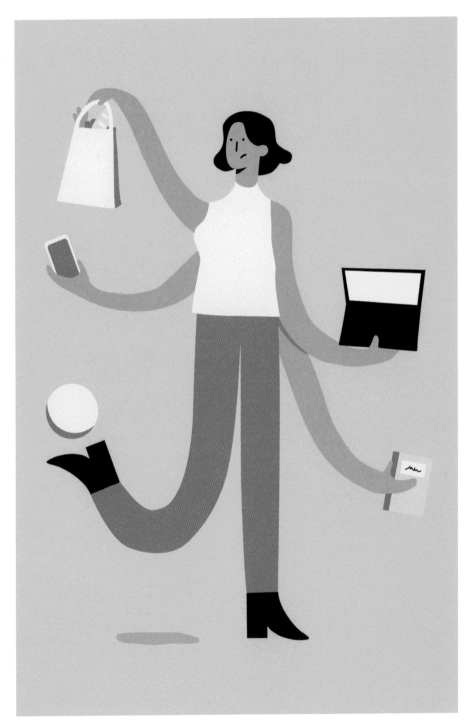

FOCUS THE MIND

IMPROVE YOUR ATTENTION SPAN

At the best of times, according to a Harvard Business School study, our attention span for a task requiring intellectual effort may be as long as 90 minutes, although it does vary from person to person. So it seems we need help here. Putting away the screens when we want to focus on something would be a good start. Our phones are not attached to our hands… Then we can also, of course, use our Sophrology tools to improve our attention span, the quality of our focus. Also, having a busy brain is not conducive to having a clear mind. If we are too busy, we may go into overload. Jane Alexander, in her book *The Overload Solution*, talks about the ten demons of overload: too much information, working too long hours, being available 24 hours a day, 7 days a week, concern about status, too much choice, looking for perfection in everything we do, change, financial difficulties, too much "stuff" and poor lifestyle. So we live in instant everything and everything goes too quickly. Let's slow down and refocus.

SHARP FOCUS ON THE ONE THING YOU ARE DOING IS THE KEY. THE RESULT WILL BE OF BETTER QUALITY AND YOU WILL SAVE ENERGY.

In fact, our brain cannot really do several things at the same time. It switches very quickly from one thing to the next when we are multitasking. This is tiring and in the end more time-consuming than doing things one after the other. And let's not even go into the quality of the results we achieve when we are multitasking: how many times have you had to start again something you tried to do while doing something else?

The key is to have a sharp focus on the one thing you are doing. The result will be of better quality and you will save energy.

So, as often as you can, do one thing at a time. As Kevin Roberts, former CEO of communications company Saatchi & Saatchi, put it:

"I am living everything to the max but slowly. Multitasking is a huge weakness. I focus on what I am doing at the time. I will give laser-like focus to this."

RELAX IN THE DOING

Although we want to focus on one thing, we don't want to drain ourselves of energy while doing so.

As I was driving on the motorway the other day, overtaking a huge lorry in my little car, I suddenly realized I was holding onto the steering wheel very tightly and my body was leaning forward as if I were trying to overtake the lorry with my body and not with my car. When I noticed, I laughed at myself and rectified my position, leaning back, breathing normally and relaxing my hands, arms and shoulders. And, guess what – I overtook the lorry just as successfully.

Have you noticed how often we do that? We put a lot of energy and physical tension into something that does not need it. We get tense as we wait for our computer to start or respond; we tighten our back muscles, shoulders and neck as we work at our desk; our whole body tenses up while we wait for something to happen… Just like when we were children and our jaws absent-mindedly munched away as we were cutting something with scissors. Perhaps, for instance, we are waiting in a queue and our body is rigid. We need *some* energy in our muscles in order to stand up without falling on the floor, but do we need that much?

If we make a habit of using twice as much energy as we need in everything we do, how much is going to be left at the end of the day?

Absent-mindedness is the key word here, I think. What we need is to be a bit more aware of what we are doing. If we sense how tense our body or part of our body is and become aware of the amount of tension or energy we actually need in order to do what we are doing, it becomes easier to relax those muscles. Hence "relax in the doing". I like that expression as it is easy to remember so that we can remind ourselves of it several times a day.

So, next time you find yourself tensing up, think about how much energy you actually need. For each item on your schedule, consider how much energy is necessary. Breathe, relax and realize how much vitality you are saving for later. It's a good way to stay bright and alert until the end of the day.

> IF WE MAKE A HABIT OF USING TWICE AS MUCH ENERGY AS WE NEED IN EVERYTHING WE DO, HOW MUCH IS GOING TO BE LEFT AT THE END OF THE DAY?

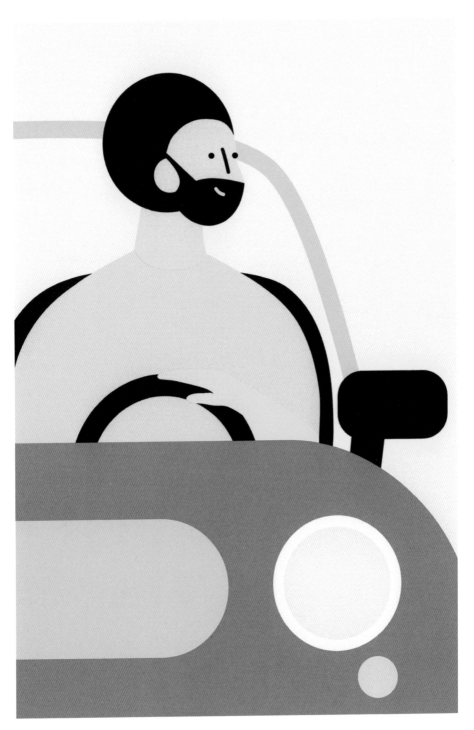

FOCUS THE MIND

MINDFULNESS

One of the core notions of mindfulness is to be fully present in whatever you are doing: aware of what your body is doing, of what you are thinking. Each time you realize your attention has slipped away, you need to bring your mind back to what you were doing or thinking.

Mindful living is both the simplest and the most complicated of tasks. Simple because it is not a very complex concept to grasp. Complicated because implementing it fully can feel like mission impossible. So my advice is: start small and build slowly from there. Great habits are not created in a day. You will probably never reach 100 per cent, but every action that is carried out mindfully will be a small victory in itself… and you will get a lot more done!

Let's go through a few ideas to get you started.

> SOPHROLOGY HELPED ME A LOT DURING A TRANSITION PERIOD, IN PARTICULAR TO UNDERSTAND HOW TO PUT THINGS INTO PERSPECTIVE AND WORK ON MYSELF, MY VALUES, MY EMOTIONS.
>
> VANESSA MAYNERIS

PRACTICAL TIPS

DIVERT ATTENTION AWAY FROM YOUR THOUGHTS

When your mind feels too full, focus on your feet – taking note of their position and how they feel – or on your breathing. You can even count your breath if that helps. This will capture your full attention, taking it away from other thoughts and refreshing the mind. Counting your breath in your head simply means you notice the normal rhythm of breathing in and breathing out. It doesn't matter whether or not your breathing is regular, whether you count slowly or quickly or for how long. It simply focuses your attention on something other than your thoughts.

BE MINDFUL IN DAILY LIFE

- Eat mindfully: what does your food taste like, look like? Notice its texture, its colours, the different smells, how it looks on the plate and what it feels like in your mouth.

- Wash the dishes mindfully: focus on what you are doing without thinking about anything else.

- Walk mindfully: think about your feet on the floor or ground; look around you and notice things.

DO ONE THING AT A TIME

As often as you can, do only one thing at a time (don't reach for your mobile phone, don't jump from one task to another, don't have several windows open on your computer at the same time, and so on).

WASH THE DISHES MINDFULLY: FOCUS ON WHAT YOU ARE DOING WITHOUT THINKING ABOUT ANYTHING ELSE.

NECK EXERCISE

Standard timing: 5 minutes

This dynamic relaxation exercise is about releasing tensions in the neck and upper back and is used here to focus your mind on a simple movement.

1. Standing up and with your eyes closed, perform the body scan described on page 20.

2. Start with a little nod of the head forward and backward, then gently and progressively make it bigger and bigger.

3. Turn your head left and right (as if saying "no"), starting with small movements and gradually moving the head further and further.

4. Make a little circle with your nose, small at first, then in a bigger and bigger spiral, as if your nose is drawing a snail from the centre outward. Do it in one direction and then the other.

5. Take a little time to listen to how you are feeling.

6. Come back into the room as described on page 20.

How do you feel? Maybe think about how you feel particularly in your neck, shoulders and upper back area. But also notice the whole body.

Feel free to record your observations in your Sophrology journal or on the notes page at the end of this chapter.

FOCUSING EXERCISE

Standard timing: 2 minutes

Like most of our dynamic relaxation exercises, this one comes directly from yoga. It is often used at the beginning of a series of Level 1 dynamic exercises as an introduction to the body scan, to put emphasis on closing our eyes and focusing inside ourselves as we do so. Here we are using it as a stand-alone practice, purely for focus, but that is the reason we don't start with a body scan .

1. Do this exercise standing up, with your eyes open.

2. Breathing in, stretch one arm out in front of you with your thumb up. Look at the thumb and focus on it. Hold your breath and bend your elbow to bring the thumb nearer your forehead. When you start to see two or more thumbs, close your eyes, touch your forehead with your thumb, then let your arm relax by your side as you breathe out.

3. You may do this just once or repeat twice more if you want.

4. Come back into the room as described on page 20.

How do you feel?

Feel free to record your observations in your Sophrology journal or on the notes page at the end of this chapter.

CLEAR YOUR HEAD

Standard timing: up to 15 minutes

Here we are using breathing to imagine we are "cleaning out" the negative feelings inside us and filling ourselves with positive energy. Breathe normally throughout.

1. Sitting down and with your eyes closed, perform the body scan described on page 20.

2. Now bring your attention to your breathing. Don't change anything, just keep breathing naturally. Then bring your attention to your head.

3. Each time you breathe out, imagine that you are letting go of tension, stress or any other unpleasant feeling, as if you were letting steam out of your body.

4. Each time you breathe in, imagine that you are physically able to bring something positive into your whole body or specifically into your head or any other part of yourself. Feel as if you are filling up with calmness, focus, clarity… whatever you feel you need.

5. Keep going for as little or as long as you like.

6. Then stop and take a short time simply to listen to your body, to how you are feeling now.

7. Come back into the room as described on page 20.

How do you feel? Any differences in the body, in the mind?

Feel free to record your observations in your Sophrology journal or on the notes page at the end of this chapter.

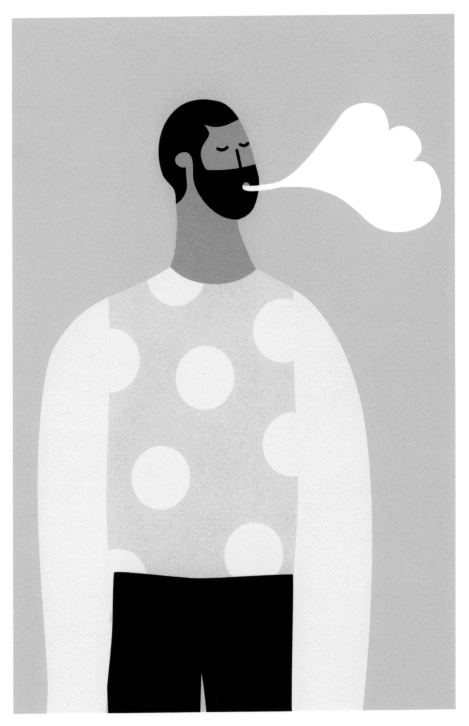

FOCUS THE MIND

PRACTISE-AT-HOME TECHNIQUES

NEUTRAL OBJECT VISUALIZATION

Standard timing: 15–20 minutes

Here you will learn how to focus on an object, a form of contemplation. But we don't use a real object; we imagine it, with eyes closed. This way, you can settle on any object that feels right for you. Be mindful, though, that we call it a "neutral" object – something simple and everyday, rather than something that has an emotional impact or a special memory attached to it. This is in order not just to learn how to focus but also to start working on non-judgment. Don't choose your object before you start – let it come to you naturally during the exercise.

Once you have found your neutral object, you can call it up any time you feel you need focus: close your eyes, recall your object, focus on it for a short while (seconds, minutes, depending on what you need), then let it go, open your eyes and refocus on what you need to do.

1. Sitting down and with your eyes closed, perform the body scan described on page 20.

2. Now let an object come to your mind – something very simple that is not attached to any particular emotion or feeling. Concentrate fully on this object, as if it is in front of your eyes and you can see it clearly. See its size, colour or colours, shape, form, texture… If possible, imagine it is rotating and you can see it from all different angles. Keep your focus – this object is the only thing you are thinking about.

3. When you feel you have done this long enough (it can be just a short time), let the image of the object go.

4. Take time simply to listen to your body, to how you are feeling now.

5. Come back into the room as described on page 20.

How do you feel?

Feel free to record your observations in your Sophrology journal or on the notes page at the end of this chapter.

ONCE YOU HAVE FOUND YOUR
NEUTRAL OBJECT, YOU CAN CALL
IT UP ANY TIME YOU FEEL YOU
NEED FOCUS.

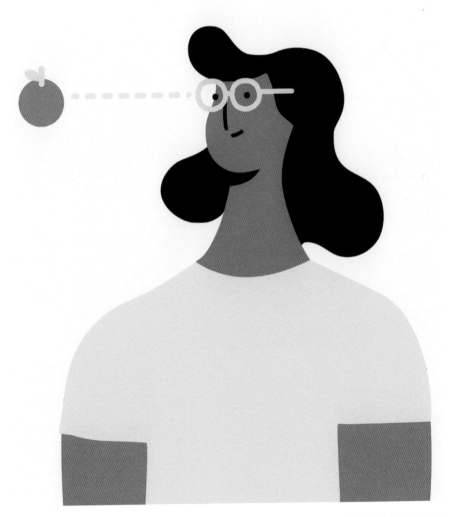

FOCUS THE MIND

OTHER TECHNIQUES
TO COMPLEMENT THIS

THE TARGET
(SEE PAGE 68)

GROUNDING: ROOTED LIKE
A TREE (SEE PAGE 121)
OR GROUNDING: BEAM OF
LIGHT (SEE PAGE 136)

SQUARE BREATHING
(SEE PAGE 109)

YOUR NOTES

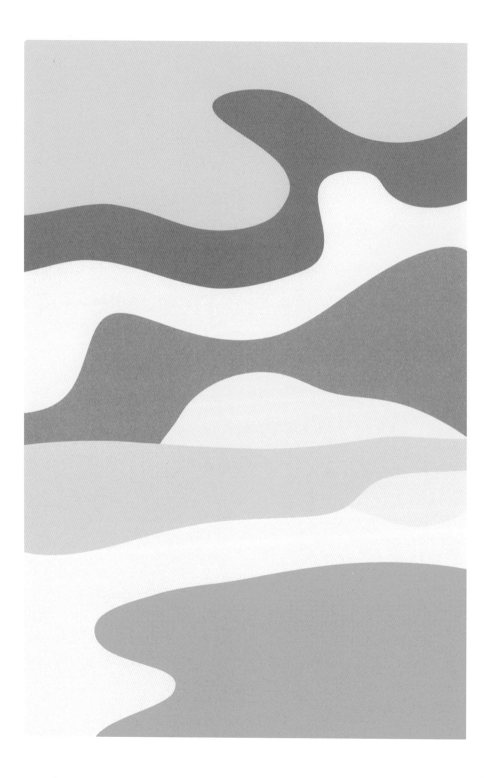

3
BUILD EMOTIONAL RESILIENCE

USING SOPHROLOGY TO ENHANCE YOUR EMOTIONAL RESILIENCE

Sophrology increases resilience. As long as you practise, of course! Let me take the marathon image again. If you think you are ready for a marathon simply because you are able to run, you are in for a big disappointment and a lot of pain on the day. You will build the stamina, the resistance, the resilience, only if you train, again and again. You can do it at your own pace, working within your own abilities, but still… you need the training.

Whatever type of exercise you are into, even if it is none at all, the marathon image works. The same would be true for a ballet dancer or for someone learning a musical instrument. Try dancing or playing without having practised regularly: your feet or your fingers will not follow what you are trying to do.

So how does Sophrology come into this? Well, whatever you do, life happens! And it will keep happening, sometimes throwing things at you left, right and centre, whether or not you practise Sophrology or any other similar technique. The difference is how you are able to react. If you are tired, emotional, mentally drained, you are not going to be in a state to react very well. In contrast, a study conducted by Dr Samantha Evans of the University of Kent on the use of Sophrology as part of an organizational change process showed that it truly helped the participants to cope with the major changes their company was going through.

> IMAGINE THAT YOU ARE LIKE A FULL GLASS OF WATER. IN SOPHROLOGY, WE WORK AT MAKING THE GLASS TOUGHER SO THAT IT CANNOT BREAK, WHATEVER STORM IS BREWING INSIDE.

Imagine that you are like a full glass of water. In Sophrology, we work at making the glass tougher so that it cannot break, whatever storm is brewing inside. Sophrology helps the mind and body react in a less intense way to a stressful situation. It reinforces the whole person, making us stronger and better able to resist life's hardships with greater serenity. People who practise Sophrology regularly say that when "something goes wrong" in their lives, they feel bad for a shorter period of time and with less intensity. In other words, they recover more quickly. They are able to handle it better. Sometimes, it can be as simple as not flying off the handle when your boss barks something at you, maintaining serenity and enough clarity to respond and manage the situation professionally while still asserting yourself. And not feeling like a wreck as a result.

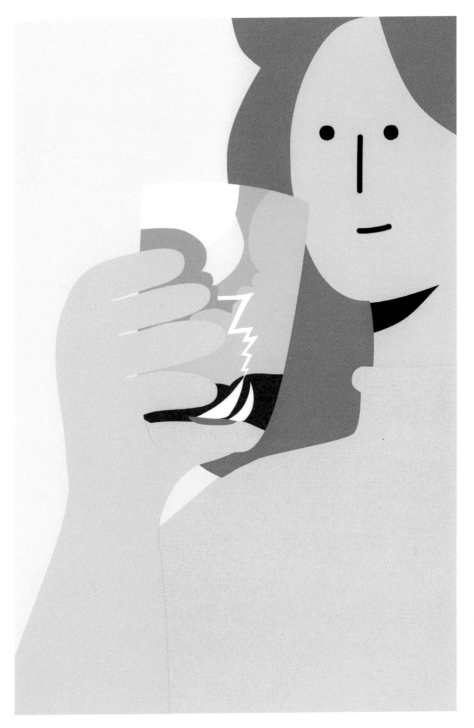

RECOGNIZING YOUR EMOTIONS

What we are talking about here is not denying our emotions and how we feel – quite the reverse. So if it is anger you are feeling toward your boss, for instance, the anger is there and is recognized. It is simply not so strong that it makes you punch that person or burst into tears. Recognizing your emotions helps you decide what to do with them. But sometimes they are still so strong that they hurt (either you or the other person… or both!). So here, we recognize the emotion, we accept it, but over time we become strong enough to deal with it in a more peaceful way. At no point in the process do we get rid of the emotion. We simply manage it differently.

In Sophrology, we say that we are trying to grow the positive inside us (remember the principle of Positive Action on page 14?), not denying and cancelling our negative feelings and emotions but putting them to one side and growing the positive to such an extent that the negative cannot have as strong a hold on us anymore: it doesn't have the space.

There are many ways to do this and the following exercises are just a few examples to get you started on the right track. All Sophrology exercises help with this in some way; here are some simple, everyday practical tips on how to approach the subject.

WE RECOGNIZE THE EMOTION AND WE ACCEPT IT. AT NO POINT IN THE PROCESS DO WE GET RID OF THE EMOTION. WE SIMPLY MANAGE IT DIFFERENTLY.

PRACTICAL TIPS

THE "POSITIVITY" BREAK

Every evening, write down three things in your Sophrology journal that have been great today, or things that have simply been nice or funny. They don't have to be anything important – the smallest things will do fine.

PUTTING ASIDE THE NEGATIVE

When starting a Sophrology exercise or whenever you are taking a break, if ideas are going round in your head about problems or difficulties you are having, imagine putting them outside the door for the duration of your exercise or break. Now focus on one happy, funny or calm thought. You can always pick the problem up at the door when you are finished.

BREATHING DEEPLY

Put your hands on your abdomen and sense how much (or how little) it moves when you breathe. This isn't a competition, so don't worry if nothing much is happening. When you breathe deeply and fill your lungs with air, your diaphragm goes down to give the lungs space, forcing your abdomen to pop out. When you then breathe out, the diaphragm goes back up and the abdominal area goes back in. So this is about playing with it, not trying too hard – noticing first how you breathe, trying to sense what, if anything, is moving, then letting your breathing become calm and maybe even slow down a little. Try gently and repeat as often as you want.

QUICK EVERYDAY TOOLS

THE TARGET

Standard timing: 5 minutes

This dynamic relaxation exercise can be used in many different ways. It can simply be a mindful, focusing exercise, allowing you to practise being present. It can also be used as I suggest here, to "punch" a particular target. In that target, you may want to put something specific that you feel like punching. It may help you release the emotion attached to the situation – or indeed to a person. (Don't worry – you are not going to punch this person in real life but it can be very helpful to admit to feelings that strong.) It can also be used when you are working on achieving a particular goal: you then place the goal in the target and put energy into the movement, but let the movement finish gently.

1. Standing up and with your eyes closed, perform the body scan described on page 20.

2. Put one foot forward and breathe in while raising your arms so that you are holding them straight out in front of you. Bend your elbow to bring the arm corresponding to your back foot in toward your shoulder, as if you are holding a bow and arrow. Hold your breath gently while focusing on an imaginary target in front of you.

3. When you need to breathe out, release your arm with your hand in a fist (as if you were releasing an arrow or punching something). Do this gently or strongly depending on what you need or can do while you breathe out through your mouth. Then let your arms fall back into place by your sides. Do this twice more, then do three times with the other side.

4. Come back into the room as described on page 20.

How do you feel?

Feel free to record your observations in your Sophrology journal or on the notes page at the end of this chapter.

CHEST BREATHING

Standard timing: 5 minutes

We are focusing here on the chest as the physical link to emotions. Do the exercise gently and be fully focused on the body, not on the emotions.

1. Standing up and with your eyes closed, perform the body scan described on page 20.

2. Close your hands into loose fists and place them on your chest, side by side. Breathe in and let your hands follow the movement as your chest opens. As you breathe out, let your hands follow the movement again, the fingers curling up as they come back to the centre of your chest. Do this simple exercise gently and slowly, focusing on the movement and the breath. Repeat three times.

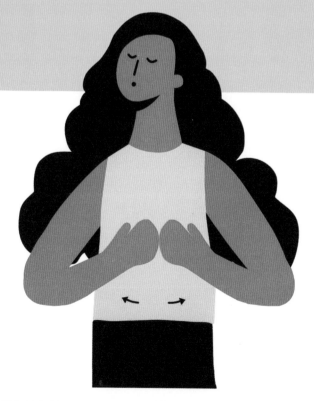

3. Take a little time to listen to how you are feeling, then come back into the room as described on page 20.

How do you feel?

Feel free to record your observations in your Sophrology journal or on the notes page at the end of this chapter.

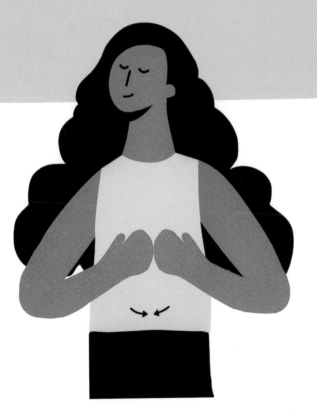

THE CUSHION

Standard timing: 5–10 minutes

With this dynamic relaxation exercise we are using a cushion to symbolically "get rid of stuff". This exercise is often used by children, but I find it works well for all ages. You can really go for it and throw the cushion at full force!

1. Standing up, with your eyes closed and holding a cushion in your hands, perform the body scan described on page 20.

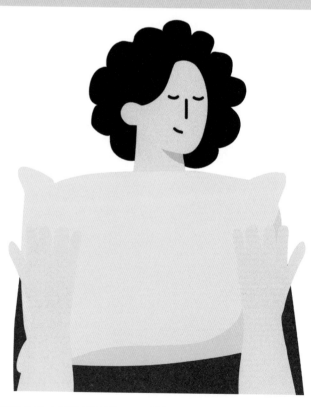

2. Imagine you are putting all your negative emotions into the cushion. These may include anger or anything else. Everything and everyone that is linked to this emotion goes into the cushion. Breathe in deeply, then breathe out loudly as you throw the cushion onto the floor.

3. Do this three times and then take a little time to listen to how you are feeling.

4. Come back into the room as described on page 20.

How do you feel?

Feel free to record your observations in your Sophrology journal or on the notes page at the end of this chapter.

PRACTISE-AT-HOME TECHNIQUES

THE BAG VISUALIZATION

Standard timing: 15–20 minutes

This is a visualization version of the cushion exercise. Here, instead of physically throwing the cushion, you imagine throwing the "stuff" away in a bag. Depending on whether you are a visual person or respond better to action, one or the other may work better for you. Try them both and see what you prefer.

1. Sitting down and with your eyes closed, perform the body scan described on page 20.

2. Imagine that you are walking along a mountain path and arrive at the foot of a mountain. On the path ahead of you, you can see a big empty bag and you decide to place in it everything you want to get rid of in your life at the moment: tensions, emotions, blocks, pains… everything you don't need at this time. You may see all these elements as images, objects, symbols, words – whatever works for you. But be aware of each and every element, know precisely what you are putting in the bag and breathe deeply and calmly as you do this.

3. Carrying the bag, you start climbing up the mountain path, looking toward your goal, the light at the top.

4. When you get there, you discover that this mountain is in fact a volcano and you decide to empty all the contents of your bag into it. You watch as the lava and flames attack everything you have thrown into them, destroying it all.

5. You descend the path with your empty bag. On the way down, you take the time to admire the landscape around you: nature, flowers, a mountain spring, birds singing, the sun shining… When you arrive at the foot of the mountain, you let all the images go.

6. Take a little time simply to listen to your body, to how you are feeling now.

7. Come back into the room as described on page 20.

How do you feel?

Feel free to record your observations in your Sophrology journal or on the notes page at the end of this chapter.

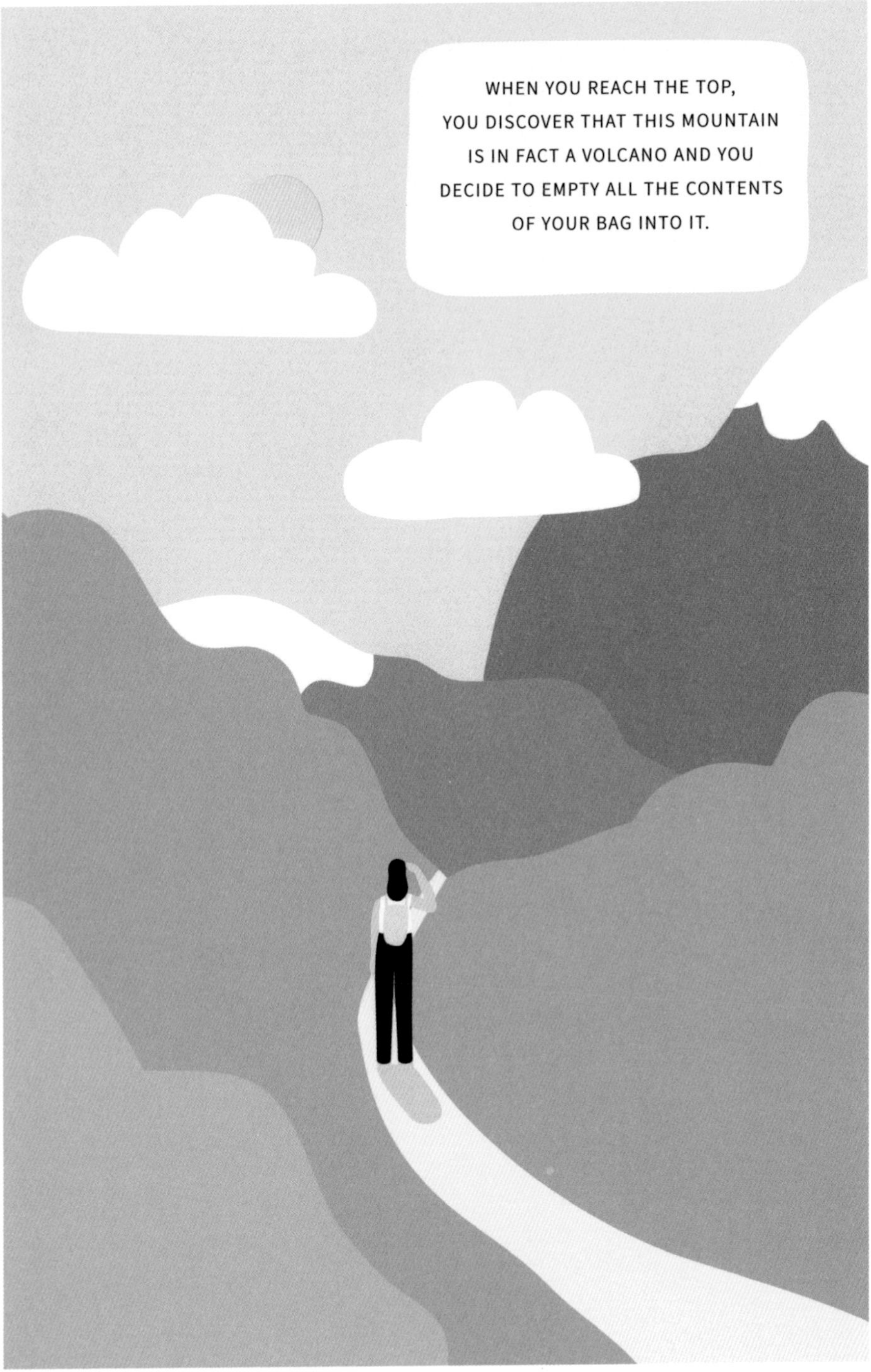
WHEN YOU REACH THE TOP,
YOU DISCOVER THAT THIS MOUNTAIN
IS IN FACT A VOLCANO AND YOU
DECIDE TO EMPTY ALL THE CONTENTS
OF YOUR BAG INTO IT.

OTHER TECHNIQUES
TO COMPLEMENT THIS

ALL DYNAMIC RELAXATION
EXERCISES (SEE PAGES 36,
38, 39, 54, 55, 88, 89, 108,
121, 136, 160, 180, 182, 197,
198) PARTICULARLY TENSE
AND RELEASE (ON PAGE 89)

YOUR NOTES

BUILD EMOTIONAL RESILIENCE

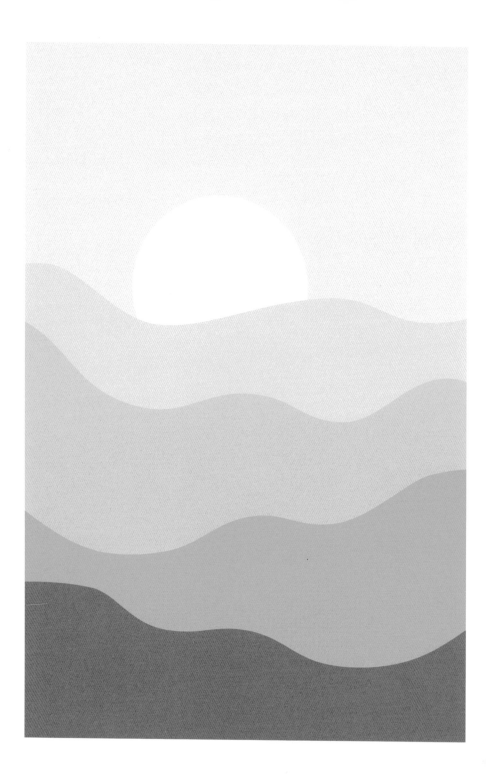

4

MANAGE STRESS & ANXIETY

STRESS, WHAT STRESS?

Let's first understand what we are talking about when we talk about stress. We have all felt stressed at one point or another, but do you really know what is happening when you feel stressed? Hans Selye, the Hungarian-Canadian scientist who first used the term in the biological sense, defined stress as a general adaptation syndrome: "the body's nonspecific response to a demand placed on it". The International Stress Management Association in the UK has also described it as "the adverse reaction people have to excessive pressures or other types of demand placed on them".

You may have heard about the "fight or flight" response mechanism: this is what happens when we are stressed.

STAGE 1

Alarm reaction. Our adrenal glands produce a shot of adrenaline, the hormone that helps us deal with stress. This is what makes us jump back if we see a car speeding toward us when we are about to cross the street. We don't need to think about it – the immediate, urgent response happens in the body.

STAGE 2

Stage of resistance. If stress continues for too long, the adrenals produce another hormone, cortisol, on top of the adrenaline to help us continue to combat the stress – for instance, to be able to keep running if that car is still coming at us.

STAGE 3

The problem is, if this continues for too long, we end up worn out, with body tensions, headaches, backaches, digestive issues, and so on. We may then reach this third stage: exhaustion, where burnout, heart attacks, strokes and other serious problems could be lurking.

The problem is not the stress itself. Stress is a perfectly natural phenomenon, but chronic and/or acute stress – or "hyper-stress" as it is now called – puts an unhealthy demand on the body. We are not meant to be under stress constantly or for periods of months or years at a time.

SIMPLIFY AND SLOW DOWN

Have you ever found yourself thinking the kettle was taking way too much time to boil or the traffic lights were too slow in turning green?

We are getting used to having everything on the spot, no waiting, no delaying, even for one second; we want instant everything.

Usually we wait until we are overwhelmed to realize that something is wrong. What if we tried to deal with this *before* that happened?

1. Do one thing at a time and be in the moment and don't juggle too many balls: put what is important in your schedule first, delegate what you can and just take things out of your timetable! Ask yourself these questions: What is vital/important/ not very important/a waste of time/draining? Where do I really make a difference and when can I delegate? What can I simply not do (learn to say no!)/do less often/ do differently?

2. Each evening, make a short list of the essential things to do tomorrow. And start with those the next day.

3. Slow down! Slowing down does not mean dragging on; it is finding the right pace for you, finding that space in your mind that will give you more space in your life.

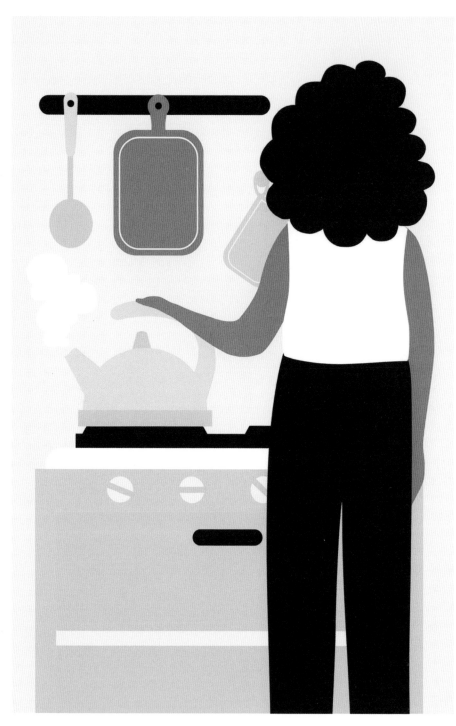

GET TO KNOW YOURSELF

Know your needs, your limits, your rhythms. Do you know how much sleep you need and at what time? Do you know when you work at your best?

Listening to what is really happening inside, letting go and relaxing is not about being weak. It is about being astute and clever, about truly knowing yourself and putting that knowledge to the best use. We tend to like that feeling of excitement produced by a rush of adrenaline and want to feel it over and over. But after a while it just masks what we are really feeling, draining us instead of energizing us, making us pretend, even to ourselves, that we are fine.

If you listen to yourself and to your body, get to know your natural rhythms, you will realize when you are at your best. It is essential to be aware of your boundaries and limits. You will also learn how to take better care of yourself in the process.

HAVE YOU EVER FOUND YOURSELF THINKING THE KETTLE WAS TAKING WAY TOO MUCH TIME TO BOIL OR THE TRAFFIC LIGHTS WERE TOO SLOW IN TURNING GREEN?

So how do you do this exactly? Well, you could start by taking time to listen to how you are feeling as often as possible during the day. And when I say take time, it will not take any time at all: it is not about stopping what you are doing, but about noticing. Notice how you feel when waking up, eating, driving, working, cooking. Pay attention to how you feel when walking outside, walking inside, arriving at work… doing anything at any point during the day, really.

Then act accordingly. Of course, if you notice that you should ideally sleep until 10am, that may not be compatible with your office hours, but perhaps you could go to bed earlier the night before? Or catch up on sleep at the weekend?

IF YOU LISTEN TO YOURSELF AND TO YOUR BODY, GET TO KNOW YOUR NATURAL RHYTHMS, YOU WILL REALIZE WHEN YOU ARE AT YOUR BEST.

Often, though, taking care of yourself is just about tweaking things a little to make a big difference to your body and state of mind. Maybe for you it is about what you eat and at what time: if that cup of tea at 3pm really perks you up, make sure you have it. Whatever it is that works for you, find it and, if you possibly can, do it.

It could also be about who you spend your time with. Notice how different people's company makes you feel. Maybe you could see more of those who make you feel positive, energized and inspired?

In Sophrology, we are big on listening to how we feel. After each exercise within a practice, we stop for a couple of minutes and listen to how we are feeling. Even if it is just to realize that our left toe is tingling or that our arms are heavy. The more we practise, the more we recognize when we are reaching our limits or starting to feel tired. We may even notice that we are about to have a panic attack before it happens, and be able to take steps to prevent it. And if we are feeling good we feel even better, because we recognize it fully and are with it 100 per cent!

> IN SOPHROLOGY, WE ARE BIG ON LISTENING TO HOW WE FEEL. AFTER EACH EXERCISE WITHIN A PRACTICE, WE STOP FOR A COUPLE OF MINUTES AND LISTEN TO HOW WE ARE FEELING.

MANAGE STRESS & ANXIETY

PRACTICAL TIPS

TAKE A DEEP BREATH

Before starting a new task, take a deep breath. What about right now? What about making sure you take at least three deep breaths every day? As we saw in the previous chapter (see page 67), most people tend not to breathe deeply enough. Breathing is important, of course, to bring oxygen to the body. And you can never have too much fuel. But also think about how the diaphragm is affected by deep breathing (see page 67): if your breathing is too shallow, the diaphragm will not move. If it does not move, it will not massage the digestive organs, the lower abdomen, the lower back, and so on. Your digestion will be disrupted. If this goes on for some time, you may experience lower back pain and many other discomforts. Stress is one of the major factors in disrupting breathing, so take a deep breath as often as you can!

LISTEN TO YOUR BODY

• While waiting for something to happen (the computer to boot up, the bus to arrive), breathe, bring your shoulders down, check there are no tensions anywhere in your body; if there are, try to let go of them.

• When walking, check whether your pace is right for you. Try changing rhythm just to notice the difference.

• Several times during the day, check in: how are you breathing? How does it feel? Does it feel right or do you want to change it?

• Listen to how you feel as often as possible: when walking, preparing a meal, switching on your computer…

SLOW DOWN, TAKE TIME

- Throughout the day, do just one thing at a time as much as possible.

- Do at least one thing more slowly than usual at some point during your day.

- Take silent moments when you need them throughout the day to check in with yourself.

- Take breaks regularly throughout the day and pay attention to how you feel.

SAVOUR AND UNWIND

- Back home, take a few minutes to unwind, doing nothing before you start anything else.

- Make mealtimes count: sit down, taste your food, savour it and enjoy it.

- Before going to bed, allow at least 30 minutes to unwind without any screen or work-related activity. Do something you love, something calm and peaceful.

QUICK EVERYDAY TOOLS

SHOULDER PUMPING

Standard timing: 5 minutes

This dynamic relaxation exercise is one of my personal favourites for stress-busting. It also gives me a lot of energy. Give it a go, moving your shoulders gently or with a lot of energy, depending of what feels right and paying attention to any pain you may have. Always be respectful of how you feel on the day.

1. Standing up and with your eyes closed, perform the body scan described on page 20.

2. Breathing in, bring your shoulders up, fists closed. Holding your breath, do an "up and down" movement with your shoulders.

Make it as brisk or as gentle as you want. When you need to, breathe out loudly and let go of shoulders, arms, hands.

3. Repeat three times.

4. Come back into the room as described on page 20.

How do you feel in your shoulders, back, whole body? Generally speaking?

Feel free to record your observations in your Sophrology journal or on the notes page at the end of this chapter.

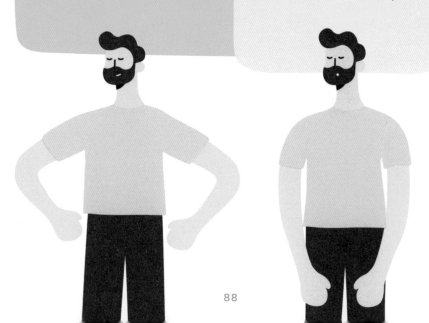

TENSE AND RELEASE

Standard timing: 15 minutes

You can practise this dynamic relaxation exercise sitting, standing or lying down. The exercise here uses all parts of the body, but you can also use just one area or skip one if something is painful. Always adapt the strength of the muscle contraction to what feels right – it can be very gentle or more intense, depending on what suits you in the moment. It is the release after the tension that is the most important thing and that reaction helps the body relax.

1. Standing up or sitting down, with your eyes closed, perform the body scan described on page 20.

2. Breathe in and gently contract the muscles in your face, sensing any tension or discomfort. Breathe out loudly, let go and completely relax the muscles, letting the tensions flow away. Do this three times and listen to how you feel inside.

3. Repeat the same thing with your neck, then with your arms, chest, abdomen, back, legs and then your whole body. Each time you breathe in, tense the muscles in the relevant area, then breathe out and relax deeply.

4. Do three times on each part of the body and three times with the whole body. Take time to listen in after you have worked on each area and again at the very end, after you have focused on the whole body.

5. Come back into the room as described on page 20.

How do you feel?

Feel free to record your observations in your Sophrology journal or on the notes page at the end of this chapter.

PRACTISE-AT-HOME TECHNIQUES

BUBBLE BREATHING

Standard timing: 10–20 minutes

This is my "signature" exercise, my personal take on a classic Sophrology practice. It was a huge help to me when I was battling burnout. The image of the bubbles can make it easier to visualize the positive and negative. Breathe naturally as you do this exercise.

1. Sitting down and with your eyes closed, perform the body scan described on page 20.

2. Now bring your attention to your breathing. Don't change anything, keep breathing naturally.

3. Each time you breathe out, imagine that a flow of dark bubbles is leaving your body, taking away the stress, tensions, anxieties...

4. Each time you breathe in, imagine that a flow of golden bubbles is coming into you, bringing in peace, calmness and quiet or anything else you may be needing at this moment.

5. Keep going for as long as feels right for you.

6. Then stop and take a little time to simply listen to your body, to how you are feeling now.

7. Come back into the room as described on page 20.

How do you feel? How easy/difficult was it to use the different-coloured bubbles? Were they leaving and coming into one part of your body in particular or the whole body?

Feel free to record your observations in your Sophrology journal or on the notes page at the end of this chapter.

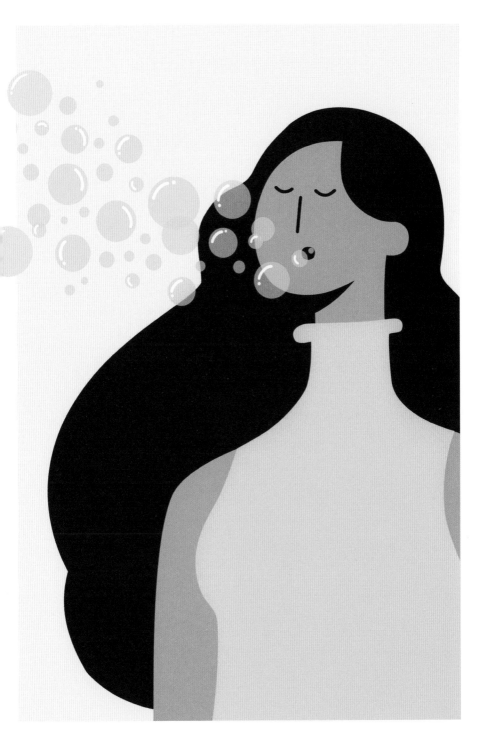

MANAGE STRESS & ANXIETY

BACK HOME VISUALIZATION

Standard timing: 15–20 minutes

**This technique is particularly useful
if you have difficulty letting go of
work stress once you are home –
thinking about it, worrying about it.
If you work from home, you can adapt
it, imagining you are closing the door
to your study for instance.**

1. Sitting down and with your eyes
   closed, perform the body scan
   described on page 20.

2. Imagine yourself leaving work.
   Picture yourself closing the door
   behind you. See the journey back
   home: the train or the car or any
   other means of transport you use.

3. Then see yourself in front of the
   door of your house or flat. Go in
   the way you usually do – inserting
   the key, ringing the doorbell or
   whatever it may be. Picture your
   entrance. Perhaps there is someone
   to greet you. Stop on the doorstep
   and have a look at what you see
   inside, the hallway, the room,
   whatever it is you see on first
   arriving home. Once you've gone
   in you choose a place in the house
   that you particularly like. You can
   see yourself choosing it, where you
   need to go to get there, the place
   you settle in, where you sit or lie
   down. Notice your body position,
   your arms, your legs. Be aware of
   how your body feels after a day's
   work. Then take a break and relax.
   Enjoy the present, being there.

4. Take a little time to listen to how
   you are feeling. Stretch, rub your
   hands and open your eyes.

How do you feel?

**Feel free to record your observations
in your Sophrology journal or on the
notes page at the end of this chapter.**

MANAGE STRESS & ANXIETY

OTHER TECHNIQUES
TO COMPLEMENT THIS

BREATHE IN THE SUNSHINE
(SEE PAGE 139)

FIVE SENSES
PRACTICAL TIP
(SEE PAGE 119)

GROUNDING: ROOTED
LIKE A TREE (SEE PAGE
121) OR GROUNDING:
BEAM OF LIGHT (SEE
PAGE 136)

YOUR NOTES

MANAGE STRESS & ANXIETY

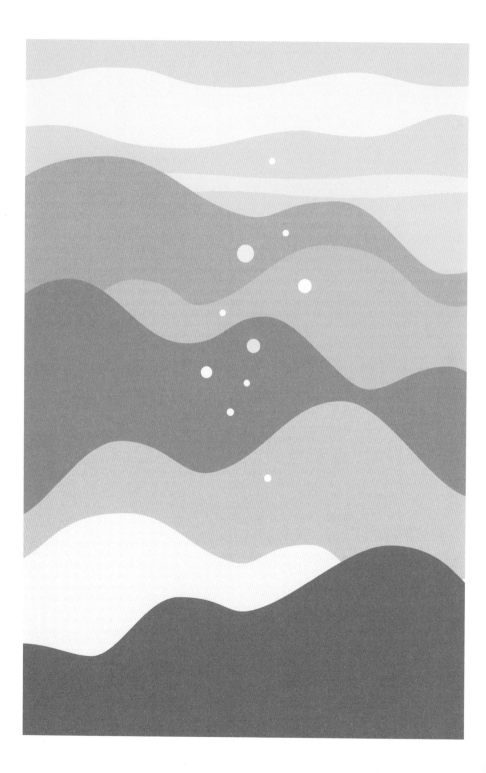

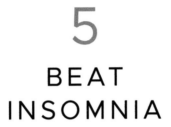

5
BEAT INSOMNIA

USING SOPHROLOGY TO IMPROVE YOUR SLEEP

The Sleep Alliance in the UK explains that "at a time when the 24/7 attitude dominates Western culture and time asleep is viewed as wasted time, many consider that a need for sleep indicates laziness or a lack of 'moral fibre'. Today's society demands a constant readiness to work and socialize, and as a result we often do not want to admit to sleepiness."

In reality, sleep is essential and we could not function properly without it. Sleep is an important part of maintaining clear brain function when we are awake. According to sleep expert Chris Idzikowski, lack of sleep will slow down your reactions and impair your thinking skills and concentration. It leads to poor memory and loss of vigilance, increased risk-taking, weight gain, depression, poor immune health, an increased risk of diabetes and morbidity, back pain and headaches, and an increased risk of early mortality.

Sleeping replenishes your energy, restores and repairs muscles and bones (for children this is when the growth hormone is released), boosts your immune system, and detoxes and renews your body. You could say sleep makes you more intelligent, being more focused and having more energy and memory.

If you have no sleeping difficulties but often feel tired or have a very full life, taking time to sleep more is probably still a good idea. Arianna Huffington, in her book *On Becoming Fearless*, set a great example in showing us how to "sleep our way to the top" – improving our performance by increasing the number of hours we sleep.

If you wish you could sleep more but have been sleeping badly for some time, a medical diagnosis is an important first step. But also Sophrology has been recommended by sleep specialists in several European countries for many years now. A study conducted by the Hôtel-Dieu Hospital in Paris in 1999 looked at its effectiveness in cases of chronic insomnia. It showed that Sophrology brought a significant decrease in sleep disorders and had a positive impact on levels of anxiety and depression. So if you are going through a bad patch or need support to complement the treatment you are already having, the exercises later in this chapter could be a good way to start.

> SLEEPING REPLENISHES YOUR ENERGY, RESTORES AND REPAIRS MUSCLES AND BONES, BOOSTS YOUR IMMUNE SYSTEM, AND DETOXES AND RENEWS YOUR BODY.

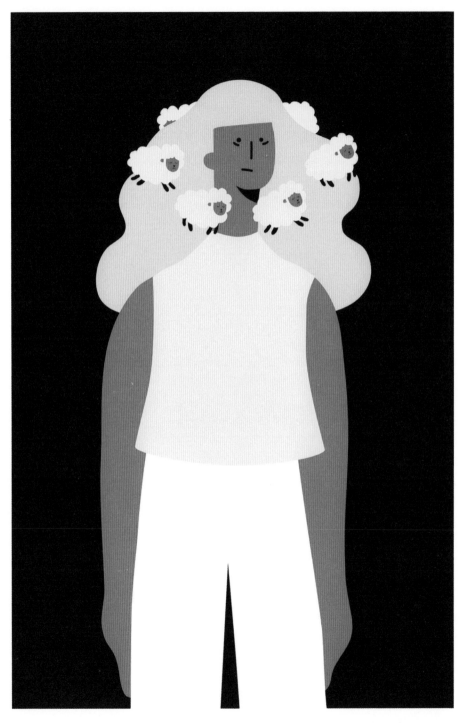

BEAT INSOMNIA

HOW SLEEP WORKS

If you have a hard time sleeping, understanding how sleep works will help you make sense of those "gaps" during the night when sleep eludes you.

We all sleep in cycles of about 90 minutes, going first into deep sleep, then into light sleep (this is when we dream) before starting another cycle. If you have difficulty sleeping you are most likely to wake up after a cycle and, if you wake up fully, find it hard to fall back to sleep before the next cycle, therefore spending the next hour and a half or so awake.

Not all cycles are of the same depth. Sleep generally gets deeper during the first half of the night and gets lighter as the hours go by, which is why a lot of us sleep quite soundly when we first go to bed and then wake up in the very early morning.

For children, sleeping is a time of general growth; for adults, it is a time when our neurons work, our brain grows and our immune system is strengthened.

It's clear we don't all need the same amount of sleep. A very small minority may feel perfectly refreshed after only five hours of sleep, some need ten. For most people, it is somewhere in between. Statistics show that some 20 years ago we slept on average eight hours a night; today the average is seven and a half hours. Over the last century we lost 20 per cent of our sleeping time. So whatever your personal needs, like most people, you are probably not sleeping enough.

The way we sleep also changes with time. Children need a lot of sleep, whereas we tend to sleep less as we grow older. It is also interesting to note that teenagers have different sleeping patterns: their need for sleep will start later at night and lead them to sleep later in the morning. This is natural and changes as they become adults. For most teenagers, the ideal time to be asleep is something like midnight to 9am, or 1am to 10am. So let them sleep late at the weekend! They genuinely need this sleep routine to help their brain and body grow.

Adults don't all have the same sleeping patterns, either: some are early birds, others feel better if they go to bed late and wake up late. Of course, work requirements don't always allow us to meet our personal needs, but staying as close as possible to your natural rhythm is the best idea.

So how do you know if you are sleeping enough? A good indication is simply that if you feel tired during the day, you are probably not getting enough sleep during the night. If you are not sure, use a holiday when you can get up and go to bed when you want to in order to assess what feels best for you. Of course, the first few days or so are probably going to be about catching up on sleep you've missed out on while you were working, but once you settle into a rhythm, make a note of it and stay as close to it as possible when you go home.

IF YOU FEEL TIRED DURING THE DAY, YOU ARE PROBABLY NOT GETTING ENOUGH SLEEP DURING THE NIGHT.

TO NAP OR NOT TO NAP?

And what about naps? Do you think taking a nap is for lazy people? Or for summer holidays under the sun? Wrong (although the holiday bit is always nice, of course!). Recent studies show that napping increases your ability to think, decreases the risk of dying from a heart attack and boosts your performance by 34 per cent.

But not just any kind of nap will do. Unless you work night shifts, a nap should always be taken between 1 and 3pm. Let's explore the different napping options.

1. The Power Nap

This is your classic 20-minute nap. If you spend more than 20 minutes, you go into deep sleep and risk feeling a bit fuzzy afterward. Keeping it to 20 minutes will boost your motor skills and alertness, helping you do a better job in the afternoon. If you are not sure you can wake up on your own after 20 minutes (it takes a bit of practice), set an alarm or ask someone to come and wake you up.

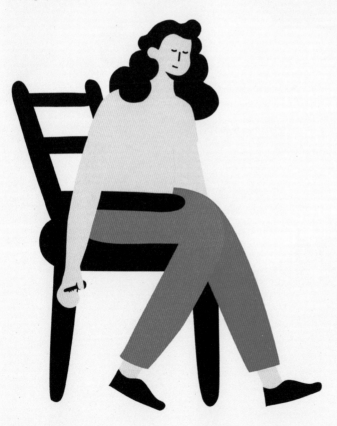

2. The Flash Nap

This was the artist Salvador Dalí's favourite. It lasts for only a few minutes, five maximum. In fact, you don't really feel as if you have slept at all. This is how he used to do it.

Sitting down on a chair, your arms hanging by your sides, hold a key between the thumb and index finger of one hand. Make sure the key will make a noise when it falls on the floor, so if you have heavy carpeting, place something like a plate under your hand. Then relax, close your eyes and imagine you are going to sleep. Let your muscles relax. When the key drops from your fingers, the noise will wake you up. This is the signal for you to stop napping and go back to work. To quote Dalí:

"You can be certain that this fleeting moment, when you have barely lost consciousness and during which you cannot be certain that you have really slept, is completely sufficient, since you will not need one more second for your entire physical and psychological being to be rested."

The flash nap is quick and easy. It is also the only nap that insomniacs can take without risking having more difficulty sleeping when bedtime comes.

3. A Longer Nap?

There are times when we are so tired we feel we could sleep for hours, at any time. Long naps are not usually recommended unless you are suffering from conditions such as an auto-immune disease, chronic fatigue, hypersensitivity or a terminal illness. Then it may be a good idea to have a nap of one or two sleep cycles – that is, one and a half to three hours – to compensate for the associated fatigue. Otherwise, stick to the flash nap or the power nap.

RECENT STUDIES SHOW THAT NAPPING INCREASES YOUR ABILITY TO THINK, DECREASES THE RISK OF DYING FROM A HEART ATTACK AND BOOSTS YOUR PERFORMANCE BY 34 PER CENT.

PRACTICAL TIPS

CONSIDER YOUR LIFESTYLE

- If you practise sports, allow at least four hours between the end of exercise and going to bed.

- Don't eat too late or too much in the evening (avoid meat, alcohol and cigarettes at night).

SET THE SCENE FOR SLEEP

- Take a warm (not hot) shower or bath (as sleep only comes when your body temperature decreases slightly). If you need help to relax before you can sleep, try adding essential oils to the bath water.

- Avoid light and noise in the bedroom. Even the smallest standby light or the fluorescent numbers on your alarm clock can halt the production of the sleep hormone melatonin.

- Be ready to go to bed when sleep comes: when you feel your eyes itching, closing, feeling heavy... go!

100%

12:57

AVOID SCREENS

- Don't keep a television, a PC or anything else with a screen in the bedroom. If you can't avoid one, cover it during the night and switch it off completely. Ideally, remove *all* electrical devices (radio, alarm clock, mobile phone…) from your bedroom, too. If you simply can't, put them at least a metre away from your head. And put the phone on flight mode.

- Don't use your mobile phone as an alarm if you can avoid it – it emits a form of low-energy radiation that is bad for your brain. If you need an alarm to wake you up, it's better to go for a traditional alarm clock. Alternatively, dawn simulators (lights that can be set to come on gradually over a period of an hour or so in the morning, so that your body responds as if to natural light) are a great option, especially if your sleep is disrupted or you find it hard to wake up. Don't look at your phone or tablet first thing in the morning, either. Don't touch any of these devices until you are fully awake and ready to go.

- See the Savour and Unwind tip on page 87. Avoid watching TV or using a computer or any kind of screen for at least 30 minutes before going to bed.

TAKE A WARM (NOT HOT) SHOWER OR BATH; SLEEP ONLY COMES WHEN YOUR BODY TEMPERATURE DECREASES SLIGHTLY.

THE WITCHING HOUR

- If you wake up during the night and feel restless: instead of tossing and turning, drink water or herbal tea, walk around calmly, breathe, read or write. Do *not* watch TV or turn on the computer and use as little light as possible. Be aware of the signs of sleep returning and go straight back to bed. If you feel better staying in bed, take the opportunity to try some of the following Sophrology exercises.

- If you are anxious about what you have to do the following day, make a list of everything before going to bed so that you are certain you will not forget anything: this should help you feel calmer. If you often find ideas coming and going and preventing you from sleeping, keep a pen and paper by your bed. You may as well download everything there and forget about them until the next morning.

QUICK EVERYDAY TOOLS

RELAXING COUNTED BREATHING

Standard timing: 5 minutes

Counting your breath here helps to create a regular rhythm to focus your mind. Try this breathing exercise if you can't sleep because you have too much going round in your head, or if you wake up in the middle of the night and are struggling to get back to sleep. Practise it while lying in bed, and do so directly, without a body scan, if you want. But bear in mind that trying it once may not be enough – give it a few goes to determine whether or not it is for you.

1. Lying down and with your eyes closed, perform the body scan described on page 20.

2. Breathe in, breathe out for a slightly longer time and then, if you can, hold your breath for a very short time when your lungs are empty. Count your breath to make it more regular and to help you focus only on your breathing and the counting, not on whatever is going round in your head. Repeat as often as you like. Don't force your breathing; find a rhythm that works comfortably for you and count at your own pace.

3. Change the rhythm if that would work better for you.

4. Take a little time to listen to how you are feeling.

How do you feel?

Feel free to record your observations the next day in your Sophrology journal or on the notes page at the end of this chapter if you fell asleep right after doing this exercise!

DON'T FORCE YOUR BREATHING;
FIND A RHYTHM THAT WORKS
COMFORTABLY FOR YOU AND COUNT
AT YOUR OWN PACE.

TENSE AND RELEASE WHILE BREATHING IN A KEY WORD

Standard timing: 5 minutes

As a preparation for this exercise, first practise the Tense and Release exercise (see page 89) during the day to get used to it, then try the Prepare for a Good Night's Sleep visualization given on page 110. At night use a combination of the two while lying in bed if you find it hard to get to sleep or wake up in the early hours, especially if you are anxious about something. Although this exercise involves breathing, it is more dynamic than most breathing exercises and, in my experience, even those who don't generally like breathing exercises enjoy this one! You can practise this exercise directly, without a body scan, if you want.

1. Lying down and with your eyes closed, perform the body scan described on page 20.

2. Breathe in and gently contract the muscles in your whole body, sensing any tension or discomfort. Breathe out loudly, let go and completely relax the muscles, letting the tensions flow away. Do this three times and listen to how you are feeling inside.

3. Then remember the key word you found in the visualization exercise. Breathe in and imagine you are breathing your word in; then breathe out and imagine it spreading everywhere. For instance, if your word is "calm", imagine you are bringing in more calmness and visualize that calmness spreading through your body, almost physically. Repeat three times.

4. Take a little time to listen to how you are feeling.

How do you feel?

Feel free to record your observations in your Sophrology journal or on the notes page at the end of this chapter. Do this the next day if you have fallen asleep by the time you finish the exercise.

SQUARE BREATHING

Standard timing: 5 minutes

When we breathe normally, we inhale, pause for a very brief moment, exhale, pause for another brief moment and then inhale again. We don't usually notice the short pauses, but they are there. Here we are expanding those pauses so that the four stages of breathing become equal in length. The idea is to give the breathing stability so that this stability will transfer to the whole self.

Try this exercise lying in bed, as soon as you realize you are waking up when you don't want to. Practise it directly, without a body scan, if you want.

1. Standing up, sitting, or lying down, and with your eyes closed, perform the body scan described on page 20.

2. Focus on your breathing and find a comfortable count that will allow you to breathe in four equal stages. For example: breathing in counting to three, waiting with your lungs full counting to three, breathing out counting to three and waiting with your lungs empty counting to three. Do this in a way that is comfortable for you, not too quickly but not too slowly either and for not too long, just the time that feels right for you. Maybe a couple of minutes.

3. Then breathe naturally again and take time to listen to how you are feeling.

4. Come back into the room as described on page 20.

How do you feel? Balanced, grounded, strong? Excellent! If, however, you are struggling or feeling anxious, swap this exercise for gentle deep breathing. Feel free to record your observations in your Sophrology journal or on the notes page at the end of this chapter.

PRACTISE-AT-HOME TECHNIQUES

PREPARE FOR A GOOD NIGHT'S SLEEP

Standard timing: 15–20 minutes

Do this visualization during the day as preparation for the exercise given on page 108. The word you use can then be recalled at night to help you fall asleep or go back to sleep.

1. Sitting down and with your eyes closed, perform the body scan described on page 20.

2. Focus on your breathing, without changing anything, just following.

3. Now imagine you are going to bed in the evening. See all the details, your usual routine, and imagine everything is going exactly as you would like. Your perfect evening, your perfect night. Imagine you are falling asleep and having an amazing, refreshing night's sleep, each breath bringing you more rest.

4. Sense how that feels. Let a word that symbolizes this restful sleep come to you. As you breathe in, imagine that you are breathing in that word.

5. Then imagine yourself waking up feeling refreshed and energized, at your best.

6. Let go of the images and come back to the present. Take a few minutes to listen to how you are feeling here and now.

7. Come back into the room as described on page 20.

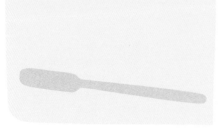

How do you feel? Have you found a word that you can use at night? If not, try a different exercise in this chapter and perhaps come back to this one another time.

Feel free to record your observations in your Sophrology journal or on the notes page at the end of this chapter.

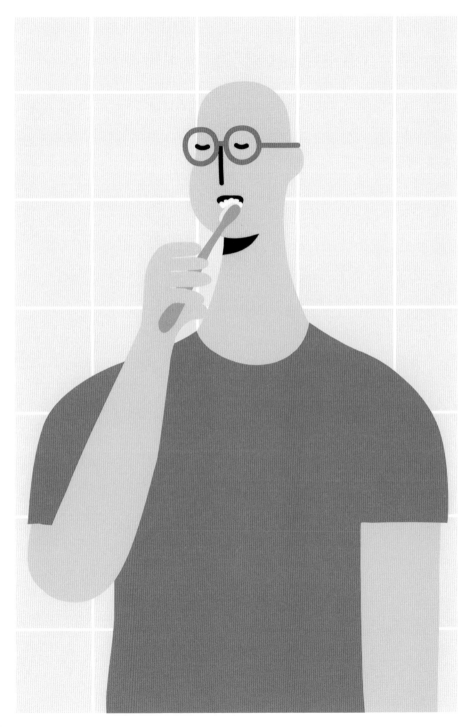

BEAT INSOMNIA

OTHER TECHNIQUES TO COMPLEMENT THIS

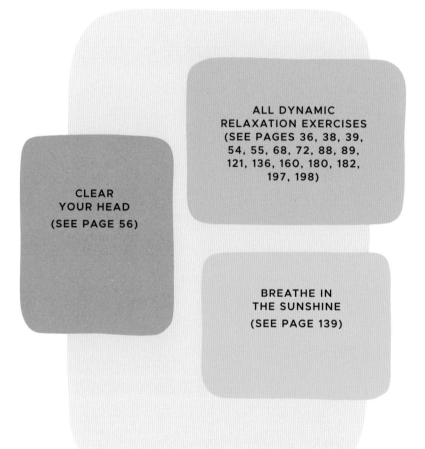

**CLEAR
YOUR HEAD**

(SEE PAGE 56)

**ALL DYNAMIC
RELAXATION EXERCISES
(SEE PAGES 36, 38, 39,
54, 55, 68, 72, 88, 89,
121, 136, 160, 180, 182,
197, 198)**

**BREATHE IN
THE SUNSHINE**

(SEE PAGE 139)

YOUR NOTES

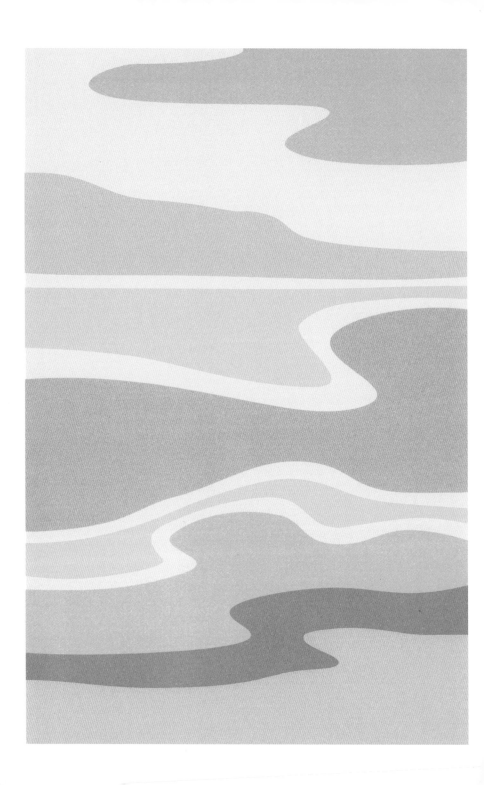

6

BOOST
SELF-CONFIDENCE

USING SOPHROLOGY
TO RAISE YOUR SELF-ESTEEM

If you are reading this chapter, you know exactly what we mean when we talk about needing more self-confidence. Whatever your issue is, whether you generally lack self-confidence or are looking for a temporary boost in one aspect of your life, such as in an interview, let's explore together how Sophrology can be of help.

If you often feel wobbly when you have to speak in a complex situation or at a particular event, the next chapter will complement this one nicely. If "wobbly" for you means physical manifestations such as shaking hands, dry throat, feeling hot and red in the face, shaky legs or anything else of that sort, you are in the right place: some of the following exercises, repeated regularly, should help you feel steadier.

If you are looking at managing a more general lack of confidence, a longer, even more repeated practice is probably what you need. Do you remember, back in Chapter 3, we talked about Sophrology enhancing emotional resilience? Here, it is more about working deep down, which in Sophrology starts with working with the body. Being in the body, finding strength inside, finding your inner power, finding also your place, your space in life. Feeling more ready from the inside for what life may throw at you.

> FLORENCE GUIDED ME STEP BY STEP TO UNDERSTAND WHAT SOPHROLOGY IS AND WHAT THIS TECHNIQUE CAN DO FOR EACH OF US IN OUR EVERYDAY LIFE. SHE OPENED A DOOR IN BOTH MY PROFESSIONAL AND PERSONAL LIFE.
>
> MARGOT ESPINASSE

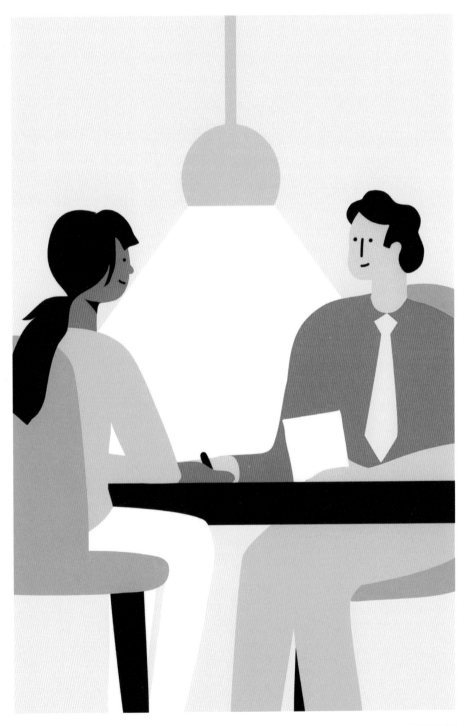

BOOST SELF-CONFIDENCE

YOUR DOUBTS ARE NOT LINKED TO YOUR ABILITIES

Remember, lack of confidence and self-doubt have nothing to do with how talented, intelligent or qualified you are. Many of the greatest stage artists felt fear all their career: Maria Callas, one of the finest sopranos of all time, apparently suffered such stage fright that she had to be literally pushed onto the stage. A well-known anecdote among theatre people tells the tale of a young actress confiding to Sarah Bernhardt that she never had stage fright, to which Bernhardt apparently promptly answered, "Don't worry, it comes with talent."

The point of these examples is that, whether it is being on stage, speaking in public or generally feeling confident in your life, your doubts are in no way linked to your abilities. There is even a phenomenon known as "impostor syndrome" – the fear of being exposed as "who you are", as someone not deserving of praise or recognition. Some of the most accomplished and successful people in the world have admitted to feeling this.

Lack of confidence can, of course, have other causes – a bad experience in the past, being in a difficult situation, fatigue and stress… But whatever the cause, we often don't know what to do about it. Being aware that it is "all in your head" does not change how you feel. Here are a few practical techniques that have been known to help public speakers, artists and many others.

> REMEMBER, LACK OF CONFIDENCE AND SELF-DOUBT HAVE NOTHING TO DO WITH HOW TALENTED, INTELLIGENT OR QUALIFIED YOU ARE.

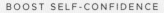

PRACTICAL TIPS

FIVE SENSES

Each day, choose one particular sense to focus on: touch, smell, hearing, taste or sight. And notice at least one thing about this sense during your day, preferably something nice. The idea is to really notice it. For instance, particularly savouring the taste of a chocolate cake, or the sight of beautiful sunshine, the perfume of a flower. Even if for only a few seconds, make a point of enjoying the experience.

POWER POSE

Imagine yourself as a Super-Hero or Super-Heroine. Wonder Woman's posture is an interesting one here – it usually makes people feel energized, grounded, powerful – but you can choose any other posture or gesture of your favourite super-hero. Strike that pose, feel the power. Use this any time you need it.

PROTECTIVE BUBBLE

Imagine yourself surrounded by a protective bubble. Not so much that you cannot communicate with the world, but enough to protect you from whatever it is that you fear. Take time to imagine it, design it (go wild!), find its texture, colour if any, thickness, size… and imagine how you "put it on" when you need it. See how you can hear, see, communicate, but sense how this could stop any negativity you don't want. Imagine how you could "take it off". And put it on any time you need it.

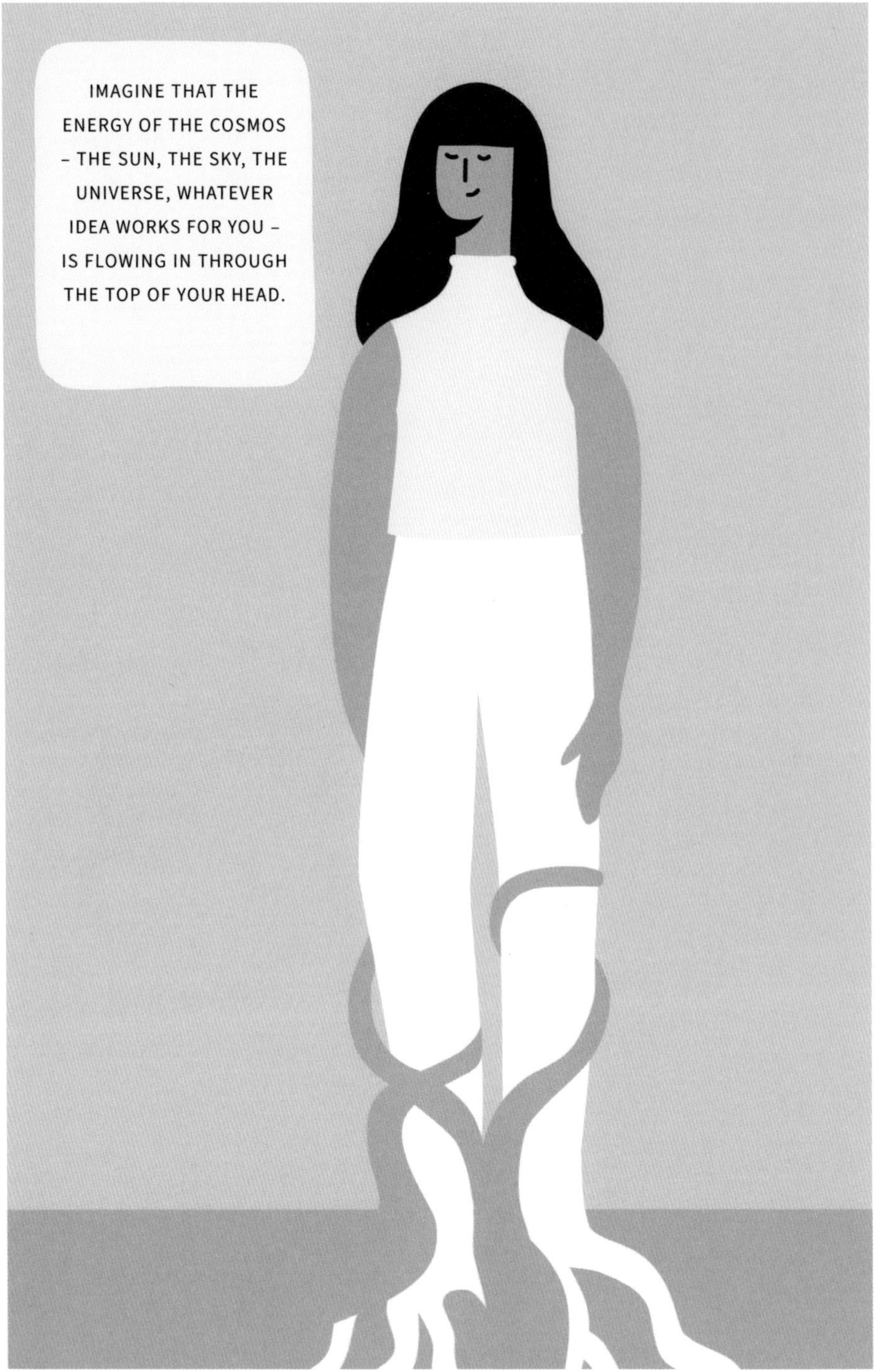
IMAGINE THAT THE ENERGY OF THE COSMOS – THE SUN, THE SKY, THE UNIVERSE, WHATEVER IDEA WORKS FOR YOU – IS FLOWING IN THROUGH THE TOP OF YOUR HEAD.

GROUNDING: ROOTED LIKE A TREE

Standard timing: 5–10 minutes

Grounding can be done in many different ways (see page 136 for a different version), so you can choose and adapt what works best for you. Ideally, do this standing up, so that you feel the energy of the position better, but if you can't stand, don't think this is not for you – try doing it sitting down, as long as your feet are touching the floor in a firm and comfortable way.

1. Standing in a relaxed and comfortable position, with your eyes closed, perform the body scan described on page 20.

2. Sense your feet firmly on the floor, noticing the parts that touch it and those that don't. Be aware of your upright position. Unclench your jaw, let your shoulders drop downward.

3. Go back to feeling your feet firmly on the floor. Sense the strength there and imagine roots like those of a tree reaching down from your feet, burrowing deep down into the earth.

4. Imagine the energy of the earth flowing up through the roots, up through all parts of your body and out through the top of your head. Allow the strong, solid energy of the earth to rise up within you.

5. Now imagine that the energy of the cosmos – the sun, the sky, the universe, whatever idea works for you – is flowing in through the top of your head, through your body and down to your feet on the floor. Feel both these flows going in different directions and mixing harmoniously in your body. Imagine this is giving you more balance, inner calmness and strength. Feel the stability within.

6. Then let the images go and take time to listen to how you feel.

7. Come back into the room as described on page 20.

How do you feel? Have you connected with the floor and/or felt interesting sensations in your legs or whole body?

Feel free to record your observations in your Sophrology journal or on the notes page at the end of this chapter.

BRING IN CONFIDENCE

Standard timing: 5–10 minutes

This breathing exercise is slightly different from those you have done so far. Up till now you have been using your natural way of breathing (apart from in the Square Breathing exercise on page 109). Here you are breathing in, then holding, then breathing out. And you are doing this only three times, whereas before you could go on for as long as you wanted. This new technique tends to make the exercise more powerful and quicker. If for some reason you are not comfortable with this format, feel free to try the same thing using your natural breathing.

1. Standing up or sitting down, with your eyes closed, perform the body scan described on page 20.

2. Using your breath, you are going to imagine you are filling yourself with more confidence. You may choose to express this simply by the word "confidence", or you may prefer to use a particular image, situation, colour or anything else that comes to mind and feels right for you.

3. Breathe in while letting the positive element come to you. Hold your breath to let it settle in. Breathing out slowly, let it spread to your whole body.

4. Repeat twice more. Always be very gentle with your breathing.

5. Then listen to how you feel.

6. Come back into the room as described on page 20.

How do you feel?

Feel free to record your observations in your Sophrology journal or on the notes page at the end of this chapter.

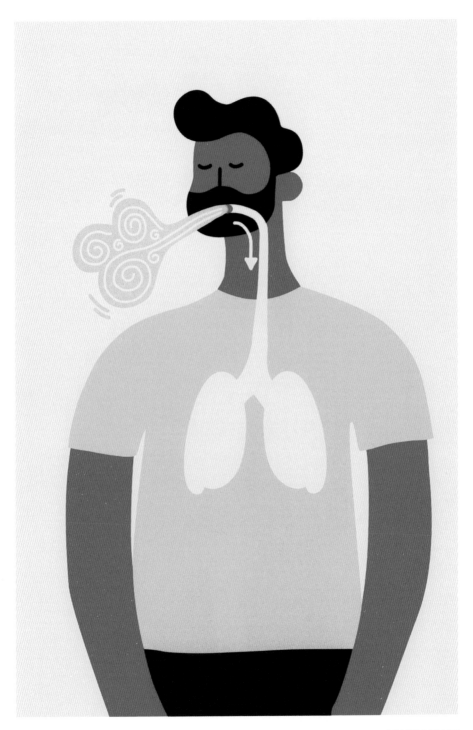

BOOST SELF-CONFIDENCE

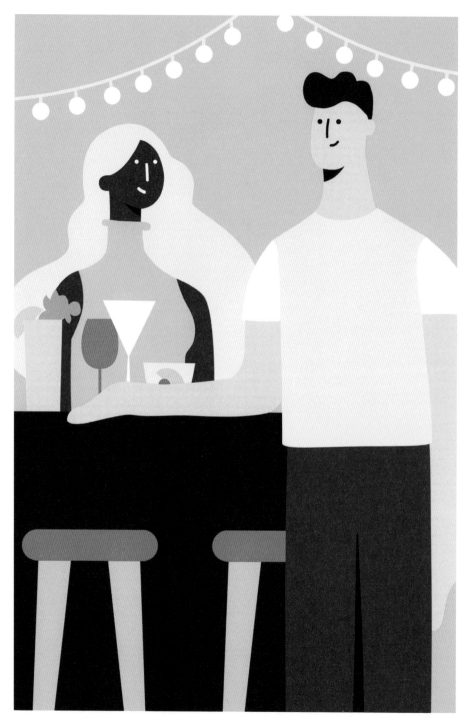

PRACTISE-AT-HOME TECHNIQUES

LOOK TO THE FUTURE

Standard timing: 15–20 minutes

For this visualization, choose an event or a moment in the future that you know is going to happen, one that is planned or organized. Choose something joyful, fun, agreeable – something that you are looking forward to. It does not have to be a big or a long thing: it could just be having a cup of tea with a friend. If you really cannot think of anything, choose something you would like to see happen. The idea is to immerse yourself in the experience, to fill yourself with the joy, peace, fun or whatever it brings you in a positive way. Then bring that portion of joy with you back to the present. This is yet another way to grow the positive feelings inside you and make you feel stronger.

1. Sitting down and with your eyes closed, perform the body scan described on page 20.

2. Imagine yourself in a situation in the future, either soon or in a while. The important thing is that you know it is planned and you are expecting it with pleasure, you know it is going to be a happy moment. It can be something very simple. It could be meeting a friend, attending a party, a joyful event…

3. Once you have this moment in mind, imagine it as clearly as possible with yourself there and everything happening just as it should. Imagine where you are and what you are doing, the colours, sounds, sights and smells around you… There may be other people there; imagine what they are saying and any other details that make it as real as possible, as if it were already happening. Let this moment fill you with its joy and any other positive sensations or emotions that are there.

4. Once you have fully enjoyed the moment, let the images go.

5. Take time to listen to how you are feeling in the here and now.

6. Come back into the room as described on page 20.

How do you feel now? How did you feel in the visualization? What was the occasion? Were you able to bring those feelings back with you? What impact has this had on you?

Feel free to record your observations in your Sophrology journal or on the notes page at the end of this chapter.

FEEL THE POWER WITHIN

Standard timing: 15–20 minutes

The idea here is to imagine yourself as being very confident in the future, and handing yourself the key to this success. The concept we are using here is that, afterward, part of you will feel as if this were feasible – in a way it will seem as if you have already "made it".

1. Sitting down and with your eyes closed, perform the body scan described on page 20.

2. Take a moment to feel your whole body from the inside, to be present in it. Also take a moment to sense the envelope, the shape, the form of your body, maybe the skin. Then your whole body, in all its dimensions. Feel your feet on the floor and breathe deeply.

THE IDEA HERE IS TO IMAGINE YOURSELF AS BEING VERY CONFIDENT IN THE FUTURE.

3. Imagine yourself in the future, at a time when you have all the confidence you feel you need at the moment. Sense what abilities and qualities you have been able to use to get to your future self. You may be able to picture this or simply to feel the strength within.

4. As you breathe in, imagine you are breathing in some of that strength, power, confidence. As you breathe out, imagine you are letting it spread throughout your body.

5. Keep all those sensations and feelings you have experienced as your future self. That energy, that success, keep them safe inside you. Know that you can find them whenever you need them.

6. Let go of all the images and take time to listen to how you are feeling in the here and now.

7. Come back into the room as described on page 20.

How do you feel? What feelings and sensations did you bring back with you? How does that affect you in the present?

Feel free to record your observations in your Sophrology journal or on the notes page at the end of this chapter.

OTHER TECHNIQUES
TO COMPLEMENT THIS

SHOULDER PUMPING
(SEE PAGE 88)

FOREARMS EXERCISE
(SEE PAGE 38)

THE PUPPET
(SEE PAGE 36)

YOUR NOTES

BOOST SELF-CONFIDENCE

7

PREPARE FOR CHALLENGING SITUATIONS

USING SOPHROLOGY TO PREPARE FOR EXAMS, INTERVIEWS & PUBLIC SPEAKING

Sophrology is often used to prepare for particular occasions: interviews, exams, driving tests, public speaking, a sports event, being on the stage, going for an operation, giving birth…The idea is not that Sophrology gives you some form of magic wand (although that would be nice, wouldn't it?). It is not a guarantee of success. It doesn't replace preparing content-wise – revising if you are taking exams, preparing answers for the most likely questions at an interview or composing a great speech if you are speaking in public. Rather, it is about enabling you to be at your best when you most need to be.

THE IDEA IS NOT THAT SOPHROLOGY GIVES YOU SOME FORM OF MAGIC WAND. IT IS ABOUT ENABLING YOU TO BE AT YOUR BEST WHEN YOU MOST NEED TO BE.

Now, of course, everyone is different, so we don't all need the same thing, but a Sophrology preparation could help with nerves as you approach most situations, and the possible sleepless nights beforehand and, of course, the moment that is usually the most difficult – just going for it.

If you suffer from nerves and anxiety, you could also refer back to Chapter 4 for advice on general stress management; if you aren't sleeping well the night(s) before, look at the sleeping advice in Chapter 5. For the rest, see the previous chapter on general confidence boosters, then look at the exercises in this chapter for more specific ideas.

If you are preparing for a particular event, don't wait until the last minute to get some support from Sophrology. Ideally, start preparing about six months before. That will give you plenty of time to work in peace and quiet, get used to the method, really integrate it into your life, repeat the exercises and choose the particular techniques that work best for you. Practise, practise, practise to build right up to the time of the event. Of course, if you don't have that much notice that this momentous occasion is going to happen and have fewer than six months left, it is still worth working on it.

A POSSIBLE SOPHROLOGY PREPARATION ROUTINE

From the previous chapters, choose the exercises that you feel you need most for stress management, better sleep and self-confidence. Feel free to add others that work for you (see the suggestions on page 142).

For the next few weeks or months, depending on how much time you have, choose at least one everyday tool per day to practise. You might like to use the same one every day for a week and then change. Once a week, choose a longer exercise.

Two or three months before your big event, start incorporating these three quick everyday tools: Grounding, Square Breathing and Breathe in the Sunshine. Perhaps focus on one for a week as you have done with the other tools. Then at the end of those three weeks, once you know these exercises and feel comfortable with them, you can practise the three of them in a row, standing, until you are able to do them fairly quickly. Once this is easy, keep practising at least three times a week. At the same time, use visualizations such as Look To the Future (see page 125) to imagine yourself in a positive future, choosing something different from what you are preparing for as the subject of the exercise.

During the last month, start experimenting with the Prepare for Success visualization on page 140. And repeat your combination of Grounding, Square Breathing and Breathe in the Sunshine tools as often as possible.

If this combination of exercises works well for you, use it just before the occasion when you have to perform, for instance in the wings if you are going on stage, while waiting for the interviewer if going to an interview, in the toilet before an exam or on public transport on your way to the big event.

> AFTER A TWO-DAY SOPHROLOGY WORKSHOP I LEARNED A SERIES OF EFFECTIVE TECHNIQUES THAT I CAN FIT IN MY EVERYDAY LIFE TO GET RID OF THE STRESS THAT WAS HOLDING ME BACK. I AM NOW FREE TO ENJOY MY WORK AND PERSONAL LIFE AND HAVE EVEN BEEN ABLE TO GO WAY BEYOND MY COMFORT ZONE WITHOUT NEGATIVE STRESS ON SEVERAL OCCASIONS.
>
> MARIE MANANDISE

PRACTICAL TIPS

BREATHE MORE DEEPLY

In Chapter 1, we talked about paying attention to your breathing, noticing how you were breathing without changing anything. Just following the pattern and speed of the breath and the places in your body that moved when you breathed. Then, in Chapter 4, I asked you to make sure you took at least three deep breaths every day. So maybe you've been trying this when you wake up in the morning or when you go to bed at night or anytime in between. How have you been getting on? Has your breathing awareness improved, has your most common breathing pattern changed?

If you feel you are now able to do this, try to let your abdomen expand as you breathe in and let it come back into place when you breathe out, maybe more slowly than you used to. If that doesn't work for you, don't force it, but if it does, it is an interesting way to breathe more deeply, to get more oxygen into your body, muscles, brain and to relax a bit more. So in the context of preparing for whatever you are preparing for, it's good for nerves!

WALK IT

As you work on your material for exams, interviews or a speech, rehearse or revise it standing up, pacing across the room, adapting your rhythm to the content, using your body to memorize or get used to what you have to say. If you can walk, out of doors, in a natural setting – whether in a forest or in a park near your home – simply go for a stroll and focus on what you want to convey in the event to come.

BREAK IT DOWN

If the whole event feels overwhelming, focus on small chunks of it at a time. Prepare for the moment just before you start; then, at another time, concentrate on the moment when you are dealing with complex matters; then move on to something else. Look at portions of it to make it less scary and prepare step by step.

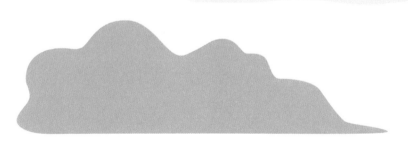

QUICK EVERYDAY TOOLS

GROUNDING: BEAM OF LIGHT

Standard timing: 10–15 minutes

This is a different take on the grounding exercise presented in the previous chapter (see page 121). Here we are focusing more on the energy aspect of it, on the strength you can take from feeling connected to the ground through that energy.

1. Standing in a relaxed and comfortable position, with your eyes closed, perform the body scan described on page 20.

2. Sense your feet firmly on the floor, noticing the parts of your feet that touch it and those that don't. Be aware of your upright position. Unclench your jaw, let your shoulders relax and drop downward.

3. Go back to feeling your feet firmly on the floor. Feel the strength there and imagine a light or colour beam or some form of energy coming from the ground through the floor.

4. Imagine the energy flowing up throughout your body and out through the top of your head. Allow the strong, solid energy of the earth to rise up within you. Breathe gently and feel the strength inside.

5. Then let the images go and take time to listen to how you feel.

6. Come back into the room as described on page 20.

How do you feel?

If you have tried this with the similar exercise in the previous chapter, how does that compare to it? Which one works better for you?

Feel free to record your observations in your Sophrology journal or on the notes page at the end of this chapter.

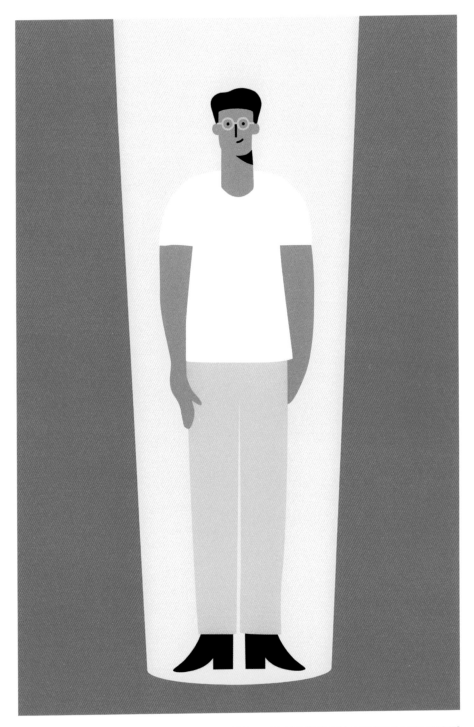

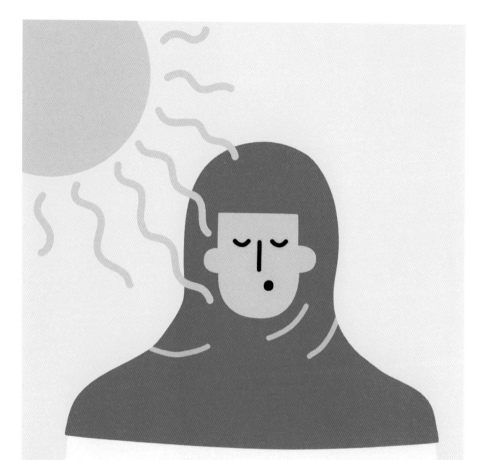

IMAGINE THAT EACH TIME
YOU BREATHE IN, YOU ARE
BREATHING IN THE SUN'S RAYS,
LIGHT, WARMTH AND ENERGY.

BREATHE IN THE SUNSHINE

Standard timing: 5–10 minutes

This exercise is about imagining you are filling yourself with sunshine and benefiting from the energy emanating from the sun. Once you know it well, you can even practise it directly with no body scan, at any moment when you feel the need for strength.

1. Standing up or sitting down, with your eyes closed, perform the body scan described on page 20.

2. Imagine you find yourself in a very sunny place.

3. Imagine that each time you breathe in you are breathing in the sun's rays, light, warmth and energy.

Let this energy, this warmth, this light into your body and, as you are breathing out, imagine it spreading everywhere, from your head to your arms, your back and your feet. Maybe there is a particular part of your body that would benefit most from it. Or go for the whole body.

4. Feel the energizing power of the sun and its warmth. Hold this visualization for a few minutes and then let it go.

5. Listen to how you are feeling. Then come back into the room as described on page 20.

How do you feel? How easy or hard was it to imagine the sunshine? Were there any specific sensations in particular parts of the body? Take time to really be with those sensations.

Feel free to record your observations in your Sophrology journal or on the notes page at the end of this chapter.

PRACTISE-AT-HOME TECHNIQUE

PREPARE FOR SUCCESS

Standard timing: 15–20 minutes

Imagining yourself in the future in a moment that you are expecting with apprehension is not easy. That is why we are choosing instead to focus on the after-event. In helping your mind to think that you have already achieved whatever it is, we give you more confidence to go for it in real life.

1. Sitting down and with your eyes closed, perform the body scan described on page 20.

2. Imagine yourself after the event you are preparing for. Maybe you are celebrating or telling friends about it. Imagine yourself recalling how you were able to do your best, be at your best, give your best. You were able to do it… How does that make you feel? Enjoy the moment, visualize the details if that works for you and know you were able to manage everything in the best possible way…

3. Then let go of the images, keep the positive feelings you may have felt and listen to how you are feeling here and now.

4. Come back into the room as described on page 20.

How do you feel? How difficult was it not to think about the event itself? Were you able to focus on the feelings of success instead? What are you taking away with you ?

Feel free to record your observations in your Sophrology journal or on the notes page at the end of this chapter.

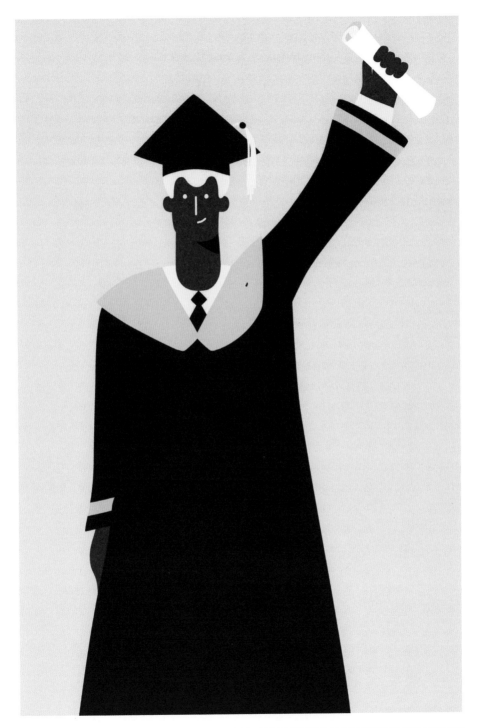

OTHER TECHNIQUES
TO COMPLEMENT THIS

SHOULDER PUMPING (SEE PAGE 88)

THE TARGET
(SEE PAGE 68)

NEUTRAL OBJECT
VISUALIZATION
(SEE PAGE 58)

YOUR NOTES

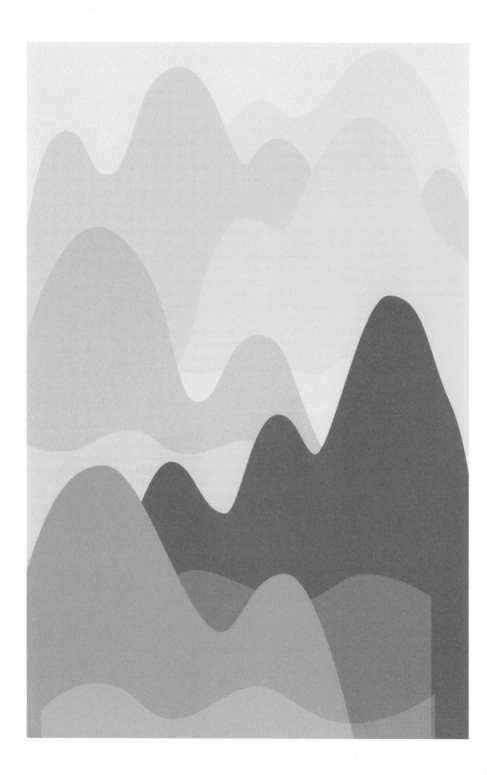

8

MAXIMIZE PERFORMANCE

In a way this is two chapters in one, because it deals with performing well at work and in the sports arena. But the exercises and techniques I recommend are the same for both – as the chapter title says, it is all about maximizing performance, whatever the context may be.

PERFORMING AT WORK

A friend of mine was told a few years ago at her work performance review that she was doing amazingly well but they were a bit worried that she did not look stressed enough… In the modern workplace, many people do seem to think that if someone is not buzzing around round the clock, they must be faking it.

Is looking super-stressed a sign of efficiency? Do you have to do everything at 100 miles an hour? Look and act super-dynamic and zoom around to show that you are the most efficient bee in the hive? Well, looking stressed and overwhelmed may impress your bosses, but it is actually very unproductive and therefore a bad idea – for you and ultimately for your company.

WHAT DOES SUCCESS MEAN?

My own experience as a super-achiever who went into burnout at the age of 23 led me to question what it means to be successful, what it takes to "get there" and how we can achieve our goals without crashing and burning in the process.

The simple fact of starting early and/or staying late at work makes us feel virtuous when in fact it is just an empty shell, devoid of any real efficiency or the reality of creating, sensing or producing.

Whether you work in an office, for yourself, from home, between several countries or in any other

way, the same seems to apply: society expects us to have a certain pattern of behaviour where "hard work" is concerned.

PEAK PERFORMANCE

Many studies show that working more than 40 hours a week decreases productivity and that if you keep doing it for more than three or four weeks, your productivity actually turns negative. Not to mention that it leads to extreme exhaustion and potential burnout.

The widely accepted Yerkes–Dodson law (named after the two psychologists who created it in 1908) says that the optimal level of stimulation for highest performance is moderate. At low levels of stimulation, a person is so disengaged and uninspired that performance flatlines; as stimulation picks up, performance strengthens, rising steadily to peak performance, but if stimulation continues to intensify, performance drops off, descending rapidly. At its most intense, the person is paralysed with stress: performance flatlines again. So we need to be challenged but not overwhelmed. At the peak of performance, we are in a state of flow. Too much going on (whether in quantity or quality) for too long and we are likely to make the wrong decision, give up or crash.

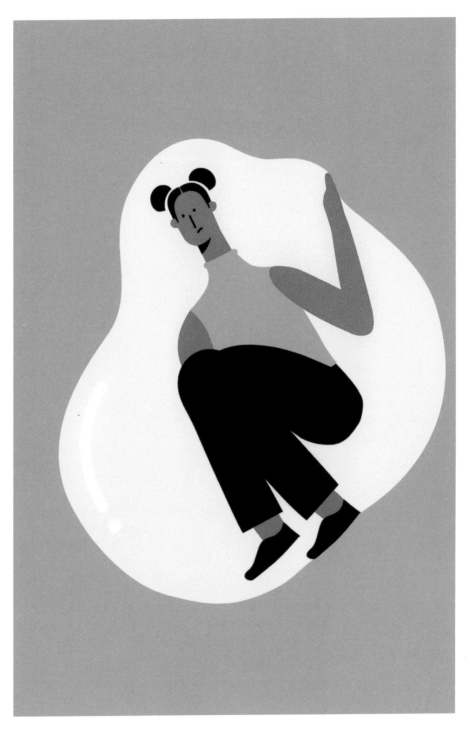

MAXIMIZE PERFORMANCE

Let's talk about what crashing can look like. Burnout is a long-term, extreme physical, mental and emotional fatigue caused by excessive and prolonged overload. You have been going through too much for too long. One day, your body switches the "off" button. In most cases, you collapse in a heap or find you are physically unable to get up in the morning. What has happened? The body has been under too much stress for too long. The adrenal glands, which produce the stress hormones adrenaline and cortisol, have been under too much pressure to perform. They end up being depleted and unable to function anymore. Hence the collapse, the burnout, the adrenal fatigue. The problem is, once this happens, you need about 12 months to recover, even if you are properly looked after. You feel unable to do anything at all – you can't work, you can't take care of the children, you can't even think clearly. You are physically, mentally and emotionally exhausted all the time. In the first months, you can barely get out of bed.

The increasing figures given in the box opposite are not accidental. We live in a world where we are expected to do more in less time and to be connected 24 hours a day, 7 days a week – and it isn't good for us.

IN THE MODERN WORKPLACE, MANY PEOPLE DO SEEM TO THINK THAT IF SOMEONE IS NOT BUZZING AROUND ROUND THE CLOCK, THEY MUST BE FAKING IT.

HOW COMMON IS BURNOUT?

- In a 2013 survey of Human Resources directors in the UK, 80 per cent said they were afraid of losing their top employees to burnout.

- Official statistics are scarce, as burnout is not officially labelled as such in many countries, but the latest estimates from the Labour Force Survey in the UK show that the total number of cases of work-related stress, depression or anxiety in 2016/17 constituted 40 per cent of all work-related illnesses.

- The latest French statistics show that 24 per cent of employees suffer from 'hyper-stress' and 12.6 per cent are at a high risk of burnout.

- In the US in 2015, more than half of physicians were experiencing professional burnout, while more recent statistics indicate that 36 per cent of those aged 18–29 and 26 per cent of those aged 30–59 often or very often experience stress and burnout symptoms.

PAUSE

This is the biggest secret to refreshing and refuelling, even when life is too full of everything: take a break, make a pause, have time off, give yourself silent times. Call it anything you want, but do it. There are many ways to do this, so let's start with a basic: the one-minute break. Unlikely as it may sound, this can recharge you for the rest of the day. It feels more refreshing to have several one-minute breaks every day than one longer one. Which does not mean that you have to skip lunch.

> "Don't just do something, sit there!"
> – Thich Nhat Hanh

In his marvellous book *The Miracle of Mindfulness*, Thich Nhat Hanh recommends a day of mindfulness and slow living every week. Not our usual weekend, is it? Most of us spend that time rushing around, doing everything we have not done during the week: shopping, housework, children's activities, "compulsory" family meals. Not to mention those of us who answer work emails from home, so that we can hit the ground running on Monday morning. As we rush through our week at 200 miles an hour, we pour everything we haven't been able to do onto the weekend and we do it at the same speed, unable to stop. But it is essential to stop. So, that one day a week of not working, not "doing stuff" – make it a priority and plan the rest of the week around it.

Because the truth of the matter is that our bodies and minds are not meant to be functioning 24/7. We are not machines. Our brains and bodies work best when they have time to recharge. When you answer your work emails from your phone at home or open your laptop to polish off a presentation, you are not working ahead. You are wasting time and energy.

On Monday morning, you will not have the fresh and clear mind that would make a difference, help you zoom through your tasks with renewed energy and find the amazing creative ideas that you need.

According to entrepreneurs Martin Bjergegaard and Jordan Milne in their amazing book *Winning Without Losing*:

> "For most of us, the 'happiness optimum' lies somewhere between 30 and 60 hours of work per week… The great tragedy is when we push ourselves past our happiness optimum in an effort to achieve success. In the process, ironically and despite our best intentions, we also pass our efficiency optimum and thus lose twice."

You also don't need to be operating at 100 per cent for everything you do. Perhaps the house doesn't need to be perfectly clean all the time. Maybe some of those emails aren't worth you spending time answering. Keep some energy for later.

WHEN YOU ANSWER YOUR WORK EMAILS FROM YOUR PHONE AT HOME OR OPEN YOUR LAPTOP TO POLISH OFF A PRESENTATION, YOU ARE NOT WORKING AHEAD. YOU ARE WASTING TIME AND ENERGY.

TECHNOLOGY & PRODUCTIVITY

We are all aware of the benefits of technology and how all those little gadgets we love so much are helping us save time and be more productive... but are they really?

While it would be next to impossible to function in the modern world without being connected to the internet (although you may want to read Susan Manshart's remarkable – and very funny – book *The Winter of Our Disconnect* on the subject), questioning the use and time spent on gadgets could lead to increased productivity. Here too, less is more.

Let's examine the facts:

Technology is robbing us of natural darkness: it is now possible to be exposed to intense light day and night. But bright screens over-stimulate our brain, keeping it awake and leading to sleeping issues. Recent research shows that even backlit tablets will decrease the level of melatonin produced, meaning that we take longer to get to sleep.

- Researcher Linda Stone has found that 80 per cent of people have what she calls "email apnea", meaning they hold their breath when an email arrives, which can contribute to stress-related diseases.

- Back in 2008, AOL's fourth annual Email Addiction Survey found that 51 percent of us checked our emails more than four times a day, 20 percent more than 10 times a day. Since then, AOL hasn't bothered to do another survey: we are now connected 24/7!

- Research from the University of London has shown that texting and emailing throughout the working day can "fog your brain" as much as smoking cannabis, knocking ten points off your IQ.

- After being interrupted at work (and how often does that happen during the day?), we need up to 25 minutes to recover our full attention and performance level.

- Studies show that if you have an electronic device at hand, your maximum focus time is... just three minutes!

And the list could go on.

BRIGHT SCREENS OVER-
STIMULATE OUR BRAIN, KEEPING
IT AWAKE AND LEADING TO
SLEEPING ISSUES.

MAKE TECHNOLOGY WORK FOR YOU

Here are some tips for avoiding technology-related stress and stopping your electronic devices taking over your life:

- Don't check your phone messages and emails first thing in the morning; give your brain and body time to wake up gently.

- As a minimum, disable the email alert on your computer; if you are feeling brave, close the email box altogether and only check your emails at set times during the day (four times maximum).

- Decide at what time in the evening you will stop checking your emails, messaging and so on – and stick to it: switch off. Make sure it is at least half an hour before you intend to go to bed.

- Turn off your mobile phone alerts (do you really need a "ping" each time someone posts a piece of trivia?) and, unless you are expecting a crucial call, disable all sounds when working on something that requires your full attention. That means switching off the vibrate mode as well!

- Step away from all your screens at regular intervals and move about: walk around the office, step outside for a while, even for a short time.

- Put your mobile phone away: in a drawer, in a cupboard, in your bag.

- Don't arrive in front of your computer or at the office without a clear list of priorities. Are you being productive or just active? Inventing things to do to avoid the important?

- Make it harder to check social media (having to go into your internet browser instead of using an app on your phone is one idea) and put a timer on how long you're on them. Allow yourself a limited time – perhaps only 30 minutes in one session.

- If you can deal with an email in two minutes maximum, do it: answer, delete, unsubscribe or delegate. Otherwise, put it in a "to read" folder or an "action" folder, not to be used as a to-do list but to be referred to when necessary.

- Introduce "switch-off Sundays" or digital detox holidays for the whole family.

SPORTS & PERFORMANCE

If you are preparing for a sporting challenge, the same principles apply as if you were trying to maximize performance in other areas of your life. If you train too little, you will not be ready and will not be at the top of your game. But if you train too much, you risk injuring yourself or even going into burnout if you are doing this at a professional level.

Most professional athletes train according to a systematic programme called periodization. This breaks training down into different phases, each focusing on a particular aspect of performance. One of its underlying principles is that phases of intense activity must be alternated with more gentle exercise and rest in order to get the best results. This means that over time you will focus on different things, depending on how long you have left before the event, but this programme can also be used if you are training for as little as a week or even a day.

You will perform better if you know when to stop, what sort of rest you need and for how long, and what other activities you need to insert in between to make it more efficient.

SOPHROLOGY FOR EXCELLENCE

So how does Sophrology fit into this, whether you are looking to perform better at work or in sports?

Dr Raymond Abrezol, the famous Swiss Sophrologist who trained so many successful Olympians, defined the ideal state of mind for those who want to achieve excellence as:

- BEING MENTALLY RELAXED -

- BEING PHYSICALLY RELAXED -

- BEING CONFIDENT
AND OPTIMISTIC -

- BEING FOCUSED ON
THE MOMENT -

- BEING FULL OF ENERGY -

- BEING MINDFUL -

- BEING IN CONTROL
OF YOURSELF -

- BEING IN YOUR OWN BUBBLE,
IN THE ZONE -

> YOU CAN USE YOUR SOPHROLOGY PRACTICE TO LEARN HOW TO RELAX, TO IMPROVE YOUR SELF-CONFIDENCE, YOUR FOCUS AND YOUR ENERGY.

This is where Sophrology comes in. You can use your Sophrology practice to learn how to relax, to improve your self-confidence, your focus and your energy. You learn to listen to yourself, to get to know yourself better so that you know when to stop, what to do when you stop in order to recharge more efficiently. You learn how to be in the zone and, in a nutshell, how to be at your best when you most need to be.

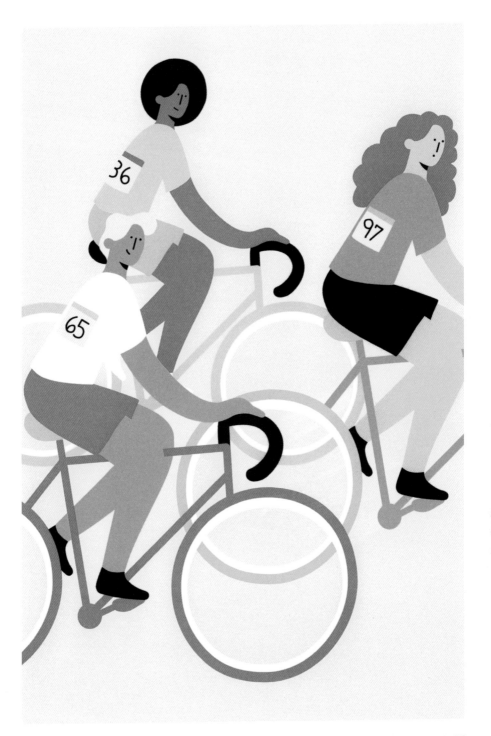

PRACTICAL TIPS

TAKE A BREAK

Several times a day, sit down, close your eyes and breathe out. Drop your shoulders, check how you feel and focus on your feet or on your breathing, without changing it, just noticing. Do this for one or two minutes maximum. But repeat it several times during the day. And rest *before* you are tired – that way, you won't need as much time to regain energy.

KNOW YOUR RHYTHMS

Keep track of how you feel when you work or train at different times of day, to find out when you are at your best for dealing with the task at hand. As much as possible, plan around what times are best for you.

WAITING = RELAXING

We owe this particularly effective phrase to Dr Luc Audouin, founder of the CEAS School of Sophrology in Paris. Whenever you are waiting for something – for the bus, for the kettle to boil or anything else – instead of impatiently moaning about how long it is taking, use the time as compulsory relaxation time.

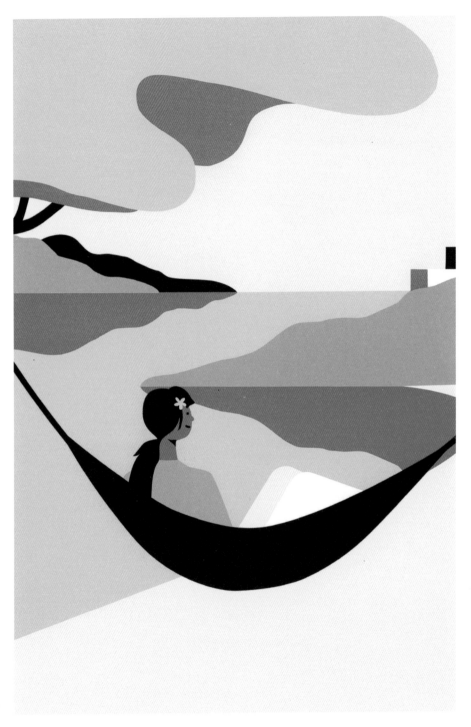

MAXIMIZE PERFORMANCE

QUICK EVERYDAY TOOLS

WHIRLING

Standard timing: 5 minutes

This is a very dynamic exercise that I recommend only if you are fit enough for it. It can be very energizing and can boost the whole body, but if you have problems with your shoulders or back, choose something gentler.

1. Standing up with your eyes closed, perform the body scan described on page 20.

2. Put one foot forward in a comfortable position and raise your arms up in front of you. Breathe in and hold your breath as you rotate the arm corresponding to your back foot forward or backward (whichever is more comfortable) in large circles. When you need to breathe out, do so and relax both arms, letting them fall back into place by your sides. Repeat twice and then do it with the other side.

3. Come back into the room as described on page 20.

How do you feel? Check that your shoulders, arms and back are feeling OK. Become aware of the sensations in your whole body.

Feel free to record your observations in your Sophrology journal or on the notes page at the end of this chapter.

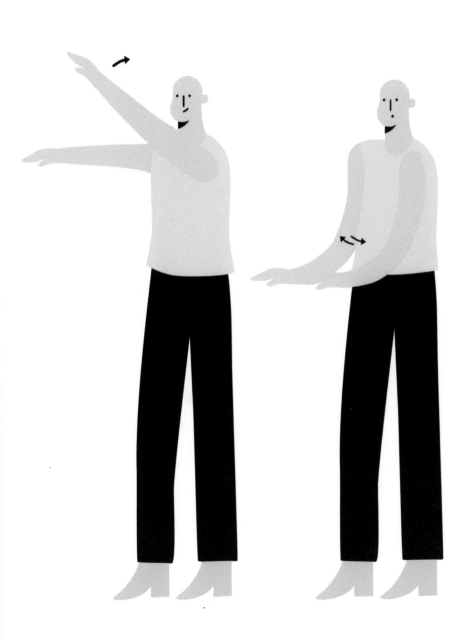

MAXIMIZE PERFORMANCE

ENERGIZING COUNTED BREATHING

Standard timing: 5 minutes maximum

This breathing exercise usually helps with energy levels, focus, and feeling very present and ready to go, all of which are on Raymond Abrezol's list of attributes for excellence (see page 156). Counting your breath here helps create a regular rhythm to make the exercise more effective and focus your mind even more. If you have difficulties with breathing exercises and/or if you are prone to anxiety or panic attacks, please discard it and use other exercises.

1. Standing up or sitting down, with your eyes closed, perform the body scan described on page 20.

2. Breathe in, hold your breath for a very short time while your lungs are full, then breathe out and start again. Count your breath to make it more regular and to help you focus only on your breathing and the counting. Don't force your breathing; find a rhythm that works comfortably for you and count at your own pace. Change the counting if that works better for you. Stop as soon as you have had enough.

3. Take a little time to listen to how you are feeling.

4. Then stretch, rub your hands and open your eyes.

How do you feel?

Feel free to record your observations in your Sophrology journal or on the notes page at the end of this chapter.

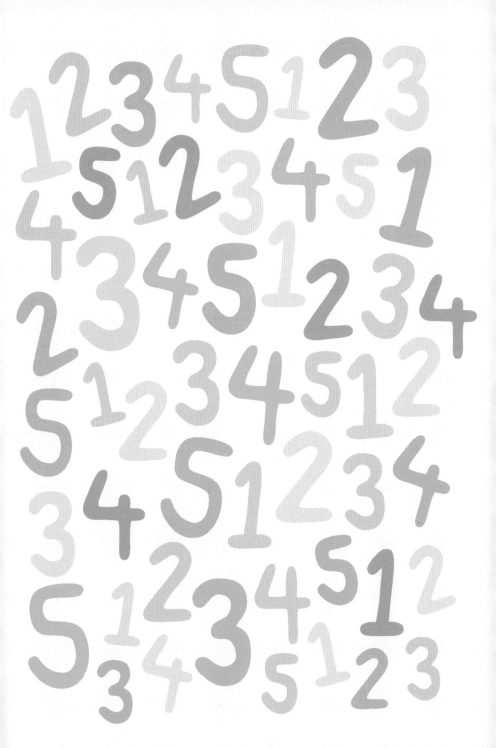

163 MAXIMIZE PERFORMANCE

LANDSCAPE VISUALIZATION

Standard timing: 15–20 minutes

This technique is about finding a safe or happy place for you to refer to when you need it. It is easier if you have good visualizing skills, but even if you don't (or if you think you don't), try it using not just your sense of sight: focus also on sounds and movements in your landscape. Whatever comes, if you feel good with this exercise, try to keep the same landscape each time you practise it so that it feels more intense and vivid. You can, of course, make additions to it (mine now has a built-in spa), but keep it generally the same. Then when you need it most, simply close your eyes and recall it (without doing a body scan first) to bring in some of that comfort, safety or whatever other positive feeling it usually gives you.

1. Sitting down with your eyes closed, perform the body scan described on page 20.

2. Let the image or idea come to you of a landscape in which you would feel good. It can be a real place that you know or an imaginary one – it doesn't matter. Try to let an image come, invite it, encourage it to emerge by itself. Welcome the first image that comes, don't discard it, as long as you feel good in it. If several images appear, wait for a little while: usually one stays longer than the others. If nothing happens, simply choose a landscape.

3. You can picture that landscape in any way you like, but see it as clearly as you can. Try to identify all the elements around you: the colours, with their different shades, brightness or softness, the shapes.

4. Maybe there are smells or perfumes or scents in this landscape. Try to smell them fully. You may also hear sounds, noises. And if you can feel yourself in this landscape, maybe you can touch something, feel the ground under your feet or the wind blowing gently on your face or the sun's rays on your skin...

5. Enjoy this moment which is all yours, like a pause, a time to relax and be comfortable. Take time to taste all its delights and how it makes you feel.

6. And now, simply let it go, let all the images go the way they came. They fade away, but you know you can find them again whenever you need them. You let them go, but you keep all the feelings you have experienced through them.

7. Take time to listen to how you are feeling here and now.

8. Come back into the room as described on page 20.

How do you feel? What are the main positive feelings you had in this landscape?

Feel free to record your observations in your Sophrology journal or on the notes page at the end of this chapter.

ANCHORING VISUALIZATION

Standard timing: 15–20 minutes

This technique is about using a simple gesture or movement that you can link to a positive feeling so that you can find that feeling again when you need it most. It is frequently used in mental preparation for sports.

Depending on what you are going to need it for (a sports challenge, some other event), choose a gesture or movement that you can use inconspicuously but not one that you could do without noticing. For example, if you wear glasses, don't use pushing your glasses back up your nose if you do that regularly. If it is for sports, perhaps a specific stretch or tapping your shoe on the floor a particular way could work. Or a simple sign with your hand. If you choose to use a pair of training shoes, for instance, or your tennis racket or golf club, make sure you have the item with you when you want to practise this exercise.

Choose your gesture before starting the exercise and also choose what you are going to use as your positive element: your landscape, maybe, if you feel great in it, or a particularly powerful memory of success, or a posture or breathing that always makes you feel good.

Practise this technique as often as you can.

In another session, you could visualize yourself using the small gesture in a future situation when you might need it.

The idea is that in the future, in an everyday situation, the small gesture will bring you back to the state of wellbeing you have linked it to. Try doing this a few times before you need it for an actual competition or challenging moment.

1. Sitting down and with your eyes closed, perform the body scan described on page 20.

2. Let the positive element you have decided to use come to you, whether it's your landscape or a positive memory or anything else that feels powerful enough for the sensations you are looking for.

3. Take time to be in or with the element and feel it as intensely as possible. As soon as the feeling is at its strongest, use the gesture or movement you have chosen, breathe in, hold your breath and anchor this feeling deep within you. Then breathe out.

4. Repeat several times if you feel like it.

5. Take time to listen to how you are feeling.

6. Come back into the room as described on page 20.

How do you feel? Was the feeling strong enough? Did you like using that gesture or do you need to find another one? If the exercise hasn't worked for you, try it again at another time. If it still doesn't work, leave it and try another tool.

Feel free to record your observations in your Sophrology journal or on the notes page at the end of this chapter.

OTHER TECHNIQUES
TO COMPLEMENT THIS

**NECK EXERCISE
(SEE PAGE 54)**

**WALKING ON THE
SPOT (SEE PAGE 39)**

**THE TARGET
(SEE PAGE 68)**

**BREATHE IN THE SUNSHINE
(SEE PAGE 139)**

YOUR NOTES

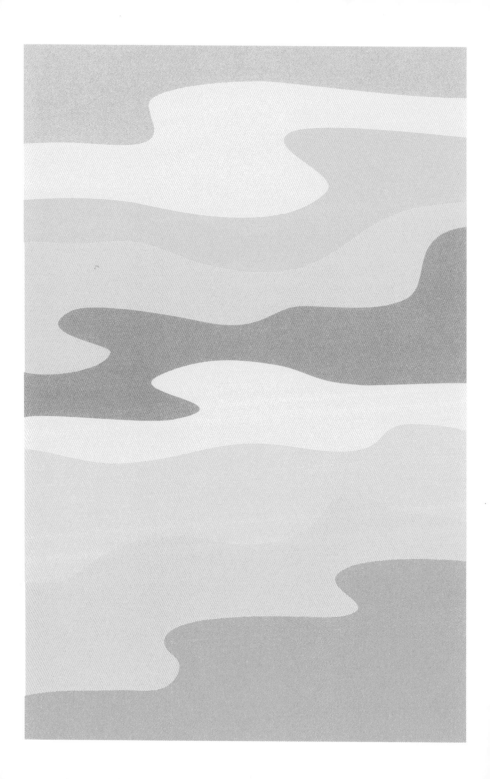

9

ENHANCE YOUR WELLBEING

USING SOPHROLOGY
TO FIND BALANCE

WORK–LIFE BALANCE

According to Martin Bjergegaard and Jordan Milne, business strategists and authors of *Winning Without Losing*:

"The most successful people have come so far exactly because they possess the skill of being relaxed in the midst of hectic activity. […] Balance is not for sissies, it is for the courageous. And it is definitely possible."

The Director of the Institute for Mindful Leadership, Janice Marturano, even goes so far as to say:

"There is no work–life balance. We have one life. What's most important is that you be awake for it."

Over the last century, our life expectancy has increased and our working hours have decreased. Do you, like me, wonder where all that "free time" has gone? Do you often feel overloaded, overwhelmed, rushing under the pressure of getting it all done?

Our timetables are so full that even the most adept organizers among us sometimes feel there is simply too much to be done.

Have you noticed, too, that what generally goes out of the window first is your personal time? The previous chapters may have given you some ideas and techniques to use in order to regain some time for yourself. Now we are going to look at putting together a proper strategy.

THE WHEEL OF LIFE TOOL

This is a useful tool for examining the various areas of your life and flagging where there may be imbalances, as a first step toward putting them right. Begin by colouring in each section (Health & Wellbeing, Career & Money, Home & Family and so on) to indicate how much time you devote to each of them at the moment, in a typical week or month. You might like to choose a different colour for each section, so that you can see the difference between them at a glance.

If you spend most of your waking time at work, or working at home, or worrying about work, colour in all of the Career & Money section – fill it to the brim! If you're spending only a couple of hours a week (or less) on Health & Wellbeing, put just a little colour near the centre of that section. If you are neglecting Relationships entirely, leave that one blank.

Look at the result. How does it make you feel?

If it all looks super-crammed and/or if any valuable sections are completely missing (like Home & Family or Personal Growth), for example, some rethinking may be in order.

Start by asking yourself, generally speaking, what makes you feel great (bearing in mind that whatever it is may not be present on your schedule at the moment)? What brings you joy? Where do you take your energy from? Make a list. If you are not sure, take a break and practise the exercise Look for Joy in the Past (see page 185) before you begin.

Look back at the chapter on stress and ask yourself the questions in it about what is vital in your schedule, what you can delegate and what you simply do not need to do (see page 81).

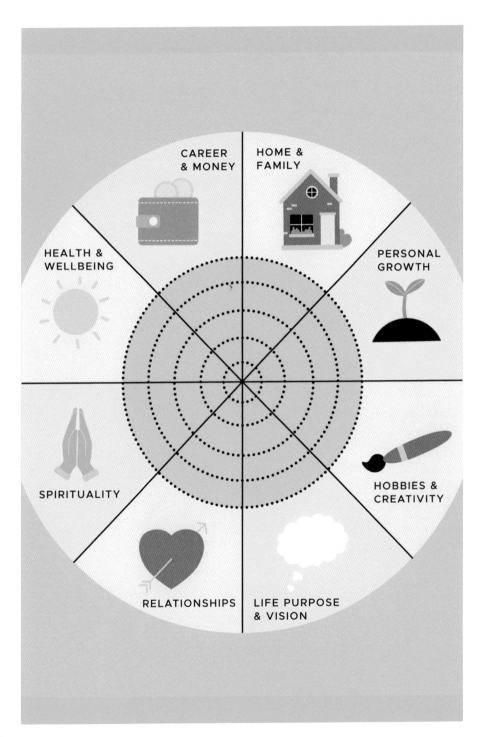

CAREER & MONEY

HOME & FAMILY

PERSONAL GROWTH

HEALTH & WELLBEING

SPIRITUALITY

HOBBIES & CREATIVITY

RELATIONSHIPS

LIFE PURPOSE & VISION

SOME FIRST AID SOLUTIONS

The idea is to put whatever is very important to you first on your schedule. You will feel better and have more energy for the rest. You could, for instance, start with putting time aside on your yearly planner for holidays. Then, on a weekly basis, assign at least one day off, really off, meant only for rest, relaxation and things that bring you joy. Reassess the rest through the vital/important/not very important/a waste of time/draining filter (see page 81).

THE DEEPER STRATEGIES

But what if, you may ask, I am already doing all these things and I still feel overwhelmed? Well, here is a secret: do less and you will be able to do more, slow down and you will arrive first. It sounds counterintuitive, doesn't it?

Our biggest mistake is to overwork, to pile up chore after chore, task after task and never to stop. Our bodies are not meant to function that way for any length of time. Our attention span, concentration levels, energy levels all need refreshing. We need to stop in order to be able to function efficiently.

At the end of the day or at the end of the week, we are exhausted; we have forgotten to take a break. Would it have been a waste of time? Quite the reverse. Only a few seconds' break can make a huge difference to your energy levels. Learning to rest and relax is essential. Life does not require all our resources all of the time – behaving as if it does is dangerous! Interestingly, the first step in going forward is to stop. Because taking a break can make a valuable difference to your levels of energy, it can improve your efficiency too.

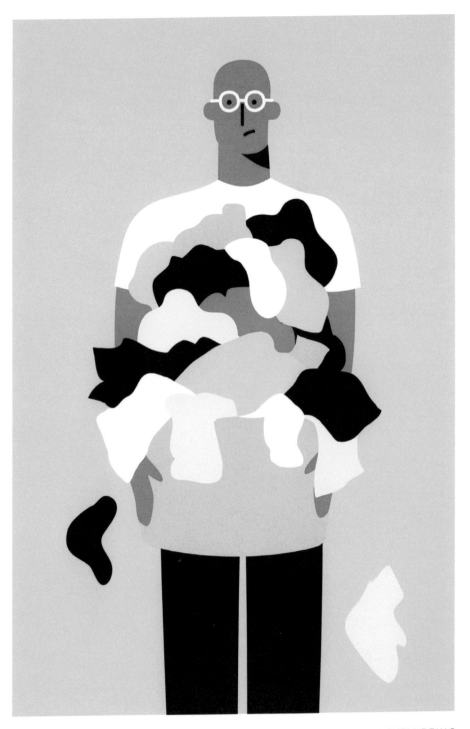

ENHANCE YOUR WELLBEING

In their book *Winning Without Losing*, Martin Bjergegaard and Jordan Milne present myriad examples of successful entrepreneurs and top executives who all have in common the fact that they have found forward-thinking ways of preserving their life balance. They quote the example of Jason Fried, founder and CEO of project-management company Basecamp, who works 40 hours a week and feels happy and balanced. He tunes into his energy levels and adapts accordingly; he is flexible and works with his body and mind instead of obeying the clock. He asks himself, "What do I feel I'd be good at right now?"

Balancing career and personal life can indeed be challenging and stressful. If you are working full time, taking care of your family, home, friends, pets… you may feel that it is mission impossible. Not everyone has the luxury of doing what they would be best at at any given moment, not everyone can choose to start working at 10am because that's what their personal energy levels and sleep pattern recommend. But there is scope for improvement and restructuring within any framework. And it is not just about making you feel good. What if the pressure is such that you end up crashing and burning? Being so driven that you forget to recharge is a huge mistake and the cost can be very high. So before you reach burnout, trying to find ways to recharge, to balance your life and keep the stress and pressure under control could be a good start. And it will keep you going a lot longer.

It also starts with taking care of yourself. Self-care: having me times, putting yourself first. For many of us, this sounds like another impossible demand. But it is not about being selfish. I have always loved the image of the oxygen masks in a plane: we are instructed to put on our own first, before helping anyone else. It took me years to fully get this. But the truth is, if you are not able to breathe, you cannot help anyone else. It is the same with life balance: if you don't take care of yourself first, you are not going to be able to take care of your family and friends or even work properly.

So, if you have not already done so, why not go back to the previous chapters and start putting together a real "feel better" programme for yourself? If you need help to get you started, use the practical tips here.

> **BEING SO DRIVEN THAT YOU FORGET TO RECHARGE IS A HUGE MISTAKE AND THE COST CAN BE VERY HIGH.**

PRACTICAL TIPS

TAKE BREAKS

Yes, to keep going you need to…
stop. I will repeat it again and again…
recharge!

As we have seen, our body and mind
are not meant to work at 100 per cent
all the time; we are not machines and
if we don't renew, we dysfunction.
After a maximum of 90 minutes, our
concentration level drops to about
zero. After too many hours of work per
week, our level of performance enters
the negative zone… So why keep at it?
High-achievers succeed this way:

- They take regular breaks (one minute
  several times a day, eyes closed).
  Remember, you need to take a break
  before you are tired.

- They use the time when they are
  waiting for something as compulsory
  relaxation time instead of getting all
  worked up.

- They have specific times with no
  connection at all to any electronic
  devices (highly recommended in the
  evenings and until you are fully ready
  in the mornings).

- They practise meditation, yoga, t'ai
  chi or Sophrology, something that
  helps them stay calm, positive and
  focused when everything around is
  a whirlwind.

LISTEN TO YOUR BODY

Is your body telling you it is tired?
Don't reach for the umpteenth cup of
coffee. Try these exercises instead: some
Square Breathing (see page 109), the
Neutral Object Visualization (see page
58), Breathe in the Sunshine (see page
139) or The Puppet (see page 36).

Your body knows best. If you listen to it
and pay attention, it will let you know
what is right.

BE MINDFUL

As we saw in Chapter 2, multitasking
is the worst idea ever. Your attention is
divided; the brain does not efficiently
do several things at the same time, it
wastes energy switching from one task
to another. Result: nothing is done as
well as it would have been if you had
given just one thing your full attention,
and working your way through your list
of tasks takes more time. So do one
thing at a time as often as possible,
focusing fully on it, not thinking about
what comes next. Enjoy the moment!

MAKE TIME FOR YOURSELF

Even and especially if you love your work, you will still tend to do too much of it. This is not a good idea if you wish to stay fresh, alert and creative. So ask yourself what renews you, what makes you feel amazing. This doesn't have to be anything complicated. It could be reading a good book, talking to a friend, watching your favourite TV show with nobody around to comment on it, taking a long bath. Don't forget to include whatever it is in your schedule, even if for only a few minutes a day. An ideal way of doing this is to put it in your diary like any other appointment. I suggest you even put it in your diary before anything else – otherwise it may never happen. To get started, schedule one "me time" each week for the next three months. Then you may feel bolder and set aside more time.

SLEEP!

We don't all need the same amount of sleep but, as we saw in Chapter 5, the vast majority of us are sleep deprived. If you often feel tired and reach for some form of stimulant during the day, there's a good chance that you are. There are some very easy ways to have better quality sleep (see the Practical Tips on page 104).

TO GET STARTED, SCHEDULE ONE "ME TIME" EACH WEEK FOR THE NEXT THREE MONTHS. THEN YOU MAY FEEL BOLDER AND SET ASIDE MORE TIME.

QUICK EVERYDAY TOOLS

SIDE STRETCHES

Standard timing: 5 minutes

Practise this dynamic relaxation exercise gently, mainly working on your presence in your body. It is not about the physical performance, stretching as far as you can go, but about being mindful of the movement. I have chosen to start with the right side to make the exercise easier to explain, but you can start with the left if you feel like it. In fact, changing the side you start on each time you do it can help increase awareness of the movement.

1. Standing up and with your eyes closed, perform the body scan described on page 20.

2. As you breathe in, shift your weight slightly onto your right foot, raise your right arm above your head and gently stretch that side of your body, keeping the other side relaxed. Keep both feet on the floor. Hold for a few seconds, then breathe out and come back to the centre. Repeat twice more on this side.

3. Come back to the centre and notice if you feel any changes between the two sides of your body.

4. Now do the same thing, three times, on your left side.

5. If you like, you can also do it one to three times with your weight evenly balanced and using both arms.

6. When you've finished, stand with your weight evenly distributed on both feet and take time to listen to how you are feeling.

7. Come back into the room as described on page 20.

How do you feel? Did you feel a difference between the two sides? A difference between stretched and relaxed?

Feel free to record your observations in your Sophrology journal or on the notes page at the end of this chapter.

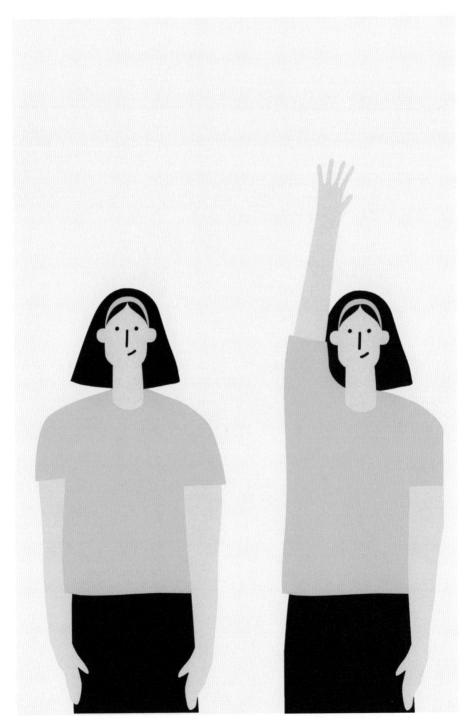

ENHANCE YOUR WELLBEING

ROTATING MOVEMENT

Standard timing: 5 minutes

Practise this dynamic relaxation exercise after Side Stretches (see page 180) to work on body awareness of both the vertical and horizontal axes and to feel the unity of your body.

1. Standing up and with your eyes closed, perform the body scan described on page 20.

2. Gently rotate your upper body from left to right, then right to left. Breathing normally, let your arms follow this movement freely, flopping around and wrapping loosely around your body as you turn. The movement can be big or small. You can do this calmly or quickly, as you like. Then let the movement stop as if by itself.

3. Take a little time to listen to how you are feeling.

4. Come back into the room as described on page 20.

How do you feel?

Feel free to record your observations in your Sophrology journal or on the notes page at the end of this chapter.

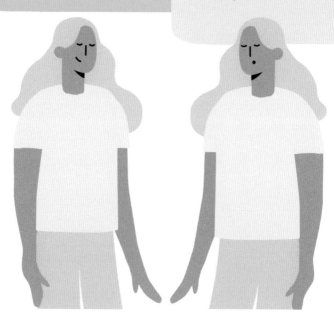

PRACTISE-AT-HOME TECHNIQUES

SUPER-CHARGED BODY AWARENESS

Standard timing: 15–20 minutes

Imagine that your body is working at its best, with your organs performing as they should. The idea is to activate the energy inside you, to sense everything working in harmony. You can imagine this in a very physical manner, thinking about your bloodstream and oxygen nourishing your body. Or you can opt for a more creative approach, imagining light or a colour flowing around inside you.

1. Sitting down and with your eyes closed, perform the body scan described on page 20.

2. Imagine the vital energy inside you increasing gently, circulating more quickly, through your whole body.

3. Start with your head, specifically your brain. Feel the energy, sensing that it is very soft, resting, nourishing.

4. Then focus on your neck and especially your thyroid. Feel the movement inside you. This warmth settling in this part of your body.

5. Now focus on your chest, lungs, heart and thymus (the gland near the base of the neck). Concentrate on the organs, imagining a gentle increase in blood circulation and temperature, bringing life and warmth, deeply reinforcing them.

6. Focus on the abdomen and digestive organs, stomach, liver, kidneys, gall bladder, pancreas, spleen, bowels. Imagine a gentle increase in blood circulation and temperature, bringing warmth and relaxation.

7. Focus on your lower body – your lower abdomen, legs and your reproductive organs. Feel the energy, sensing that it is very soft, restful and nourishing.

8. Focus on the whole body and all your organs; imagine them gently activated (from the brain to the perineum), a bit warmer, more energetic, more fully alive. Unified, working together in harmony, the whole body as one.

9. Take time to pause and listen to how you are feeling.

10. Come back into the room as described on page 20.

How do you feel?

Feel free to record your observations in your Sophrology journal or on the notes page at the end of this chapter.

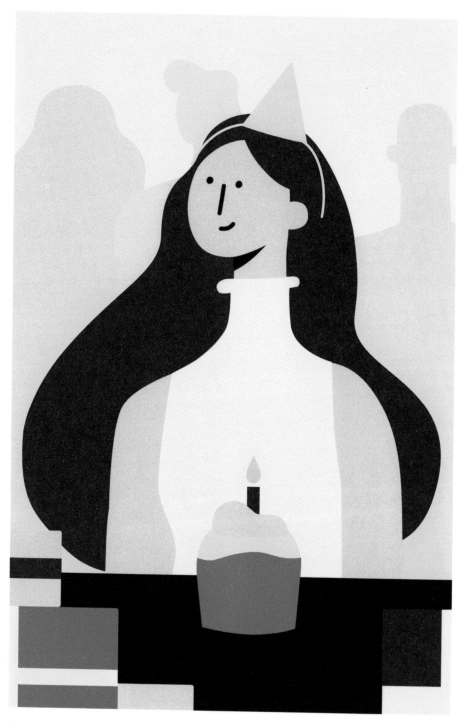

LOOK FOR JOY IN THE PAST

Standard timing: 15 minutes

Feeling good, balanced and joyful is not a given when life is tough. But fortunately most of us do know what a good moment feels like.

Here we are looking for the memory of such a moment, the more powerful the better. Again, we are growing the positive inside ourselves, step by step, exercise after exercise.

1. Sitting down with your eyes closed, perform the body scan described on page 20.

2. Remember a time or times when you were doing something that made you feel great, joyful, really happy. Maybe something that gave you lots of energy. When you felt yourself. Maybe it is a hobby that you have forgotten about or not done much of recently, maybe an aspect of your work that you are good at and enjoy, even if it is very simple. Maybe it is something mundane that you had forgotten how well it makes you feel. It could be something recent or a long way back in time, big or small, it doesn't matter. If several things come, explore them one after the other.

3. Whatever it is, remember it in as much detail as possible, look for the environment, the context, shapes, colours, sounds… and be particularly attentive to how it made you feel.

4. If something negative appears, breathe out gently and imagine you are replacing it with calmness. And look for something more positive.

5. For each memory, retain how it made you feel and let go of the images that appeared. Once you have finished the exercise, you might like to make a list of the elements you want to remember.

6. Now take time to listen to how you are feeling here and now.

7. Come back into the room as described on page 20.

How do you feel? What are you bringing back with you to use in the future?

Feel free to record your observations in your Sophrology journal or on the notes page at the end of this chapter.

OTHER TECHNIQUES
TO COMPLEMENT THIS

THE PUPPET (SEE PAGE 36)

WALKING ON THE
SPOT (SEE PAGE 39)

BUBBLE BREATHING
(SEE PAGE 90)

GROUNDING: ROOTED LIKE
A TREE (SEE PAGE 121) OR
GROUNDING: BEAM OF LIGHT
(SEE PAGE 136)

BREATHE IN THE SUNSHINE
(SEE PAGE 139)

LANDSCAPE
VISUALIZATION
(SEE PAGE 164)

YOUR NOTES

ENHANCE YOUR WELLBEING

10

REACH YOUR
TRUE POTENTIAL

USING SOPHROLOGY TO REALIZE YOUR POTENTIAL

You may be thinking that Sophrology provides a lot of simple tools for everyday difficulties and you would, of course, be right. But there is also a lot more to it than that. If you practise regularly and over a period of time, you usually come to notice some changes in the way you approach life. Perhaps you feel more relaxed about it in general, perhaps more resilient, as we have already discussed. Practised this often, Sophrology can also help you to explore your life purpose and to build a positive future for yourself.

"If we are not aware that we are happy, we are not really happy."
– Thich Nhat Hanh

BEING MORE TRULY YOURSELF

We have already covered quite a lot of ground together and if you have put all this into practice, well done! Maybe you have already noticed some changes in your life, in the way you approach things or how you react. I am sometimes reminded of how much my reactions have changed through 25 years of practising Sophrology.

My daughter pointed it out the other day when I told her how my son had broken a small plate I really liked that could not be replaced. I simply asked if he had hurt himself and helped him clear up the mess… end of story. She recalled the huge crisis that had happened nearly 20 years before when she had broken a favourite vase of mine. Tears, screams, something very close to a toddler's tantrum… on my part! For me this illustrated very well the change within. I also feel I have become more able to understand myself, live positively and express who I truly am and to take action to get where I want to go.

Here are a few well-tested techniques to get you there on your own path.

I AM SOMETIMES REMINDED OF HOW MUCH MY REACTIONS HAVE CHANGED THROUGH 25 YEARS OF PRACTISING SOPHROLOGY.

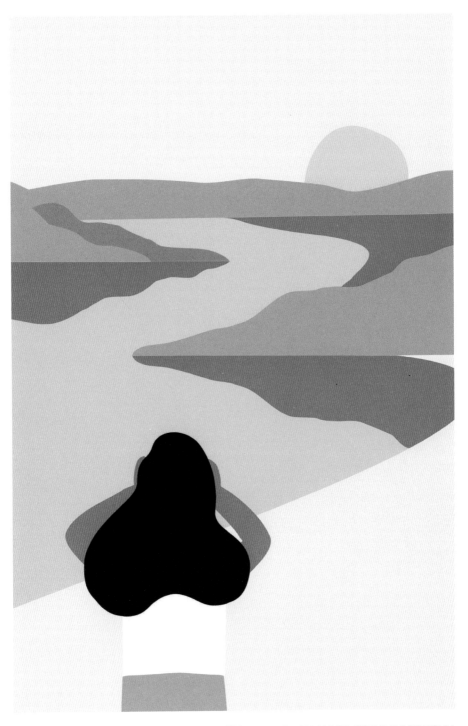

REACH YOUR TRUE POTENTIAL

NOTICE HOW YOU FEEL

Remember that in Sophrology we listen at the end of each exercise to notice how we feel. You will have tried it several times already if you have been practising the exercises in this book. I wonder how you got on with it. Some people find it hard at first to notice anything. That is perfectly OK – don't worry, just keep trying. Remember: practise, practise, practise, it's the art of repetition. The idea is that the more you practise listening in on yourself, the better you become at knowing how you feel (and that is how you *really* feel, not just "fine, thank you!"), and what you truly want. It may even feel scary at first but it's so worth it, don't you think?

BE PRESENT IN YOUR LIFE

Live it to the full, be aware, don't just drift in it, letting the hours go by aimlessly, one after another. Notice even the simplest things, enjoy them. And even something that is not very enjoyable may have some silver lining to it. (I'm not talking about something downright insufferable – leave that!) As we have seen several times in this book, be mindful, as often and as much as possible, in everything you do.

THE MORE YOU PRACTISE LISTENING IN
ON YOURSELF, THE BETTER YOU BECOME
AT KNOWING HOW YOU FEEL

SLOW DOWN

It may take a while to grasp the concept of slowing down in order to get there quicker, but seriously, get started on this one, it could revolutionize your life. Sometimes we need to act quickly, of course, to avoid a car accident or catch something before it falls. But rushing through writing a report is not going to make it of better quality, nor give you the right energy to do everything else you have to do afterward. Start with trying to walk differently, slightly more slowly. And breathe first before doing anything. See what happens!

SIMPLIFY

We tend to make everything more complicated than it needs to be, often because we feel rushed, so we go ahead quickly without giving something enough thought first (see Slow Down, the previous technique). Here the thing to do is stop, pause, breathe, think! We might be able to drop some things from our schedule entirely, without even noticing. Always ask yourself, "What if this was not completed in time or not done at all or…?" to give it perspective. If something does have to be done, find what is really important about it, the core of it. How do you get there in the simplest way possible? Now you can get started. This is a bit like decluttering your whole life, not just your wardrobe. I am a big fan of *The Minimalists* (www.theminimalists. com) on this subject: if you have not seen their work, have a look – it is a good way to start with the material aspect of things before applying the technique to your whole life.

PRACTICAL TIPS

TAKE TIME TO DO… NOTHING!

Shocking concept, isn't it?

You should have seen my children's faces the first time they told me they were bored and I answered it was good for them.

We tend to be always doing, doing, doing. Schedule times in your diary to do nothing. It's an important way to avoid wearing yourself out – and so to help you to achieve your full potential.

BE IN SILENCE

This may not be the easiest advice to follow if you work in an open-plan office and have three screaming children at home. But that is actually when you need it most. Schedule and plan it if there is no other way, perhaps telling your colleagues or family you will be on voicemail for an hour, but do it regularly. If it feels scary, start small, maybe ten minutes in the park with no phone, no music. When you feel ready, step up and eventually you may find yourself booking a three-day silent retreat.

LISTEN IN

To fulfil your true potential and be truly yourself, you need to know who you are. Take time for yourself, be in silence… and listen in. To me, this is the most important aspect of Sophrology and if you keep just one thing from this book, I hope it will be this one: take time to listen in to how you are feeling. It may start with feeling tingling in your arms, but it may well end up with enabling you to connect deeply with who you truly are.

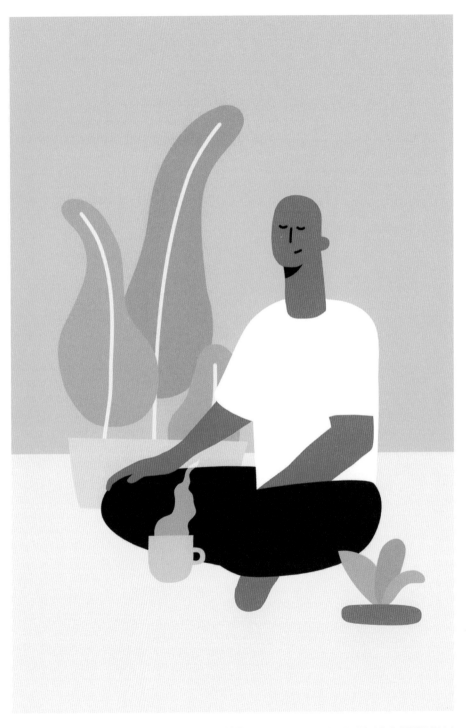

QUICK EVERYDAY TOOLS

CAPACITIES VISUALIZATION

In Sophrology, capacities means what you are capable of, your qualities, abilities… Most of us tend not to reach our full potential. This exercise is designed to help.

1. Every evening, before going to bed, take a moment to pause, close your eyes, breathe and focus on something you did really well that day, even a small thing.

2. Then think of something that perhaps you could have done better. What capacity would have helped you there – self-confidence, strength, empathy? Think of a time when perhaps you demonstrated that capacity in the past.

3. Remember how that felt and take a moment to let it sink in.

DYNAMIC RELAXATION

Standard timing: See individual exercises

I have put together for you here a list of the dynamic relaxation exercises we have seen in this book in their logical order (from head to toe). I suggest that you include some of these in your own programme to practise regularly. You can of course mix and match, but doing several of them in a row with just a few moments of silence to listen in after each one will help deepen your practice.

Focusing Exercise (see page 55)

Body Scan (see page 20)

Neck Exercise (see page 54)

Shoulder Pumping (see page 88)

Chest Breathing (see page 70)

The Target (see page 68)

Forearms Exercise (see page 38)

Side Stretches (see page 180)

Rotating Movement (see page 182)

Walking on the Spot (see page 39)

The Puppet (see page 36)

FOUR SIDES BODY AWARENESS

Standard timing: 5 minutes

This dynamic relaxation exercise is about becoming more aware of your body as one, of yourself as a whole, inside out, discovering who you are in an unusual way, maybe discovering new things about yourself.

1. Lie down on your back and notice the way you make contact with the floor. Turn over onto your right side and become aware of the changes. Discover your whole side, how you are breathing in that position, the imprint you would leave on the floor if it were sand.

2. Turn over again and, if it is not uncomfortable, lie on your stomach. Sense the changes here, too.

3. Turn onto your left side. Sense all the points where you are in contact with the floor, noticing how everything is placed.

4. Turn one last time, so you are lying on your back again. Feel your whole body coming together as a unit, from head to toe, as if you are putting together the pieces of a jigsaw puzzle.

5. Come back into the room as described on page 20.

How do you feel?

Feel free to record your observations in your Sophrology journal or on the notes page at the end of this chapter.

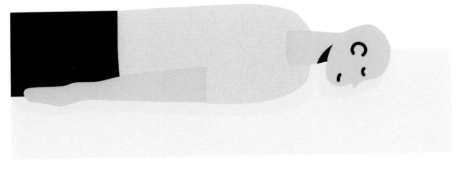

PRACTISE-AT-HOME TECHNIQUES

MINDFUL WALKING

Standard timing: as long as you like

The emphasis of this dynamic relaxation exercise is on coming back to your own natural rhythms, to following your own pace and focusing your attention inside as well as outside, on who you are in the world.

1. Go for a walk outside – in a park or the countryside or simply around the block. You can also do this exercise at a time when you are walking to somewhere specific, as long as you are not in a hurry.

2. Find your own rhythm, what works for you: if it is a quick pace because that is what you need today, that is fine. But be aware of what your mind needs and follow that lead.

3. Notice your steps, the way your feet come in contact with the ground, how your whole body feels and the way you are breathing. You could also notice your surroundings: the colours, maybe birds, plants and interesting buildings. Always do so in relation to how you feel.

When back home, feel free to write in your Sophrology journal – or on the notes page at the end of this chapter – how you felt and what you discovered on your walk.

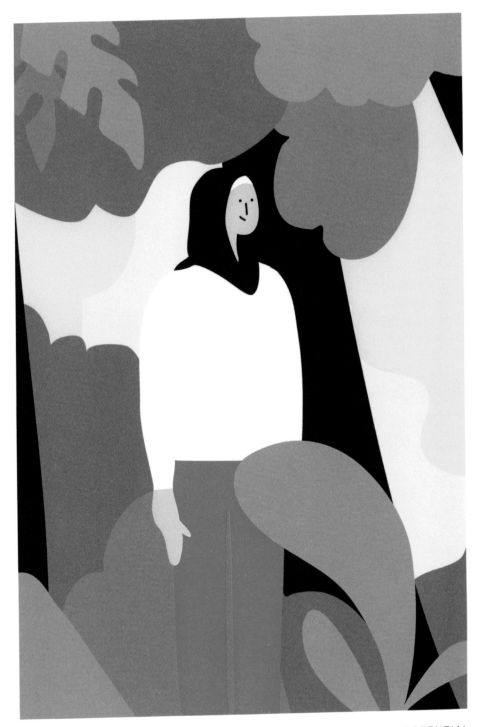

REACH YOUR TRUE POTENTIAL

DISCOVER YOUR LIFE VALUES

Standard timing: 15 minutes

We all have values that guide our lives. Not moral values, but personal values.Something that is important for each of us. For instance, family may be particularly important for you, or work, freedom or achievement. Or many other things – the list is endless. These are the things that make you tick and, if they are not respected, you may feel that you are being attacked or criticized. So it is important to know what they are. Your values may also change as you evolve over time. In this exercise, we look at what is essential for you that you may want to focus on even more forcefully in your life. You can repeat the exercise as often as you need to and use it to explore as many values as you want to each time you do it.

1. Standing up or sitting down, with your eyes closed, perform the body scan described on page 20.

2. Take time to let a value appear that is essential to you. Something that gives meaning to your life, that is perhaps a cornerstone of it or that you feel should be. Reflect on it for a while. How important is it for you? Is that importance reflected in your present life and, if so, how? When you are focusing on it in your life, how does that make you feel?

3. As you breathe in, let your arms come up above your head in a wide V shape with your head slightly tilted back (if that is not painful) and imagine you are letting this value express itself. Then breathe out and let your arms come back down to their original position by your sides. As your hands pass in front of your body, imagine you are filling yourself even more with this important value.

4. Sit back down and meditate on the presence of the value in you.

5. If you like, repeat the exercise with another value.

6. Then take time to listen to how you are feeling here and now.

7. Come back into the room as described on page 20.

How do you feel?

What value have you worked on? Record in your Sophrology journal – or on the notes page at the end of this chapter – its importance and the reflections and sensations attached to it in the exercise. Has this practice perhaps brought some light to a situation you are going through at the moment? How could it be better expressed in your life in the future?

WE ALL HAVE VALUES THAT GUIDE
OUR LIVES. NOT MORAL VALUES,
BUT PERSONAL VALUES.

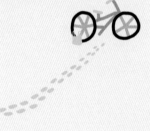

OTHER TECHNIQUES
TO COMPLEMENT THIS

FEEL THE POWER WITHIN
(SEE PAGE 126)

PREPARE
FOR SUCCESS
(SEE PAGE 140)

LOOK FOR
JOY IN THE PAST
(SEE PAGE 185)

SUPER-CHARGED BODY
AWARENESS (SEE PAGE 183)

YOUR NOTES

REACH YOUR TRUE POTENTIAL

CONCLUSION

I hope you have enjoyed discovering Sophrology in my company. Perhaps you have put together your own personalized programme to really get to know it. As we have seen, Sophrology is all about practice: you can read any number of books on the subject but you will not truly understand it until you have tried it.

As a final thought, you might like to know my personal daily routine with Sophrology. I always do a minimum of ten minutes in the morning and ten minutes in the evening.

• In the morning I do a combination of four dynamic relaxation exercises. I tend to rotate these according to what I need most or what issues in my life I am working on at that moment. Then I add either a breathing exercise or a short visualization – I have a great fondness for Bubble Breathing (see page 90), which is my own take on a popular Sophrology exercise. Then I finish with a long time of silence and listening in.

• In the evening, before going to sleep, I focus more on breathing and simply being.

But we are all different, so I do urge you to find your own Sophrology routine, keep referring back to the book for help – and enjoy life!

REFERENCES & RESOURCES

Books

Abrezol, Raymond. *La Quête de l'Excellence* (Fernand Lanore, 2013).

Alexander, Jane. *The Overload Solution* (Piatkus, 2007).

Audouin, Luc. *Bien dans son corps au quotidien* (Editions d'Organisation, 2003).

Bjergegaard, Martin & Milne, Jordan. *Winning Without Losing* (Profile Books, 2014).

Carr, Nicholas. *The Shallows* (W W Norton, 2010).

Dement, William C & Vaughan, Christopher. *The Promise of Sleep* (Dell, 2000).

Esposito, Richard et al. *Guide de Sophrologie Appliquée* (Elsevier Masson, 2017).

Evans, Samantha. *Sophrology, Organisational Change and Employee Well-being* (Project Report, Kent Business School, 2016).

Freud, Michèle. *Réconcilier l'Ame et le Corps* (Albin Michel, 2007).

Gautier, Pascal. *Découvrir la Sophrologie* (InterEditions, 2011).

Herrigel, Eugen. *Zen in the Art of Archery* (Routledge & Kegan Paul, 1953).

Huffington, Arianna. *On Becoming Fearless* (Little, Brown, 2007).

Idzikowski, Chris. *Sound Asleep* (Watkins, 2013).

Jamelot-Bonnaillie, Anne. *How can moving my shoulders up and down help me get more out of life?* (Light Bubble, 2017).

Jamison, Christopher. *Finding Sanctuary* (Liturgical Press, 2007).

Manshart, Susan. *The Winter of Our Disconnect* (Profile, 2012).

Nhat Hanh, Thich. *Peace Is in Every Step* (Rider, 1991).

Nhat Hanh, Thich. *The Miracle of Mindfulness* (Beacon Press, 1975).

Servan-Schreiber, Florence. *3 Kifs par jour* (Marabout, 2014).

Soojung-Kim Pang, Alex. *Rest* (Basic, 2016).

Magazine

Sophrologie, Pratiques et Perspectives.

Websites

https://www.theminimalists.com

ISMA (International Stress Management Association UK): https://isma.org.uk

Useful References

The statistics relating to burnout given in Chapter 8 come from Robert Half UK (February 2013): *HSE – Work-related Stress, Depression or Anxiety Statistics in Great Britain* (2017); *Observatoire du Stress au Travail Stimulus* (2017); *Technologia* (2013–17); the Mayo Clinic 2015; and *Statista* 2017.

Linda Stone's work on "email apnea" (Chapter 8) is discussed at https://lindastone.net

Sophrology Organizations

International Sophrology Federation https://sophrologyinternational.org

In the UK:

The Sophrology Network
http:/thesophrologynetwork.co.uk

In France:

Syndicat des Sophrologues Professionnels
https://www.syndicat-sophrologues-professionnels.fr

In Belgium:

Association Européenne de Sophrologie Dynamique
https://www.sophro.be

How to Find a Sophrologist

https://sophrologyinternational.org/find-a-sophrologist

http://www.sophroacademy.co.uk/sophrologists-directory

http://thesophrologynetwork.co.uk/members

http://feps-sophrologie.fr/annuaire.html

Where to Study to Become a Sophrologist

http://www.sophroacademy.co.uk

http://feps-sophrologie.fr

INDEX

ACKNOWLEDGMENTS

For this book and my whole Sophrology journey, thanks go to my teachers, Luc and Luce Audouin, Monique Cabeza and all the others along the way, a path which is never over as I keep learning every step of it.

To the very first Sophrologist I worked with, you changed my life!

To all those who followed, my colleagues, my students, thanks for everything.

To my family and friends for their support.

To Arnaud, Fabienne, Ingrid, Vincent, Maeva, Aurelie, Alexia, Isa, Liz and Audrey, who are making it possible for me to bring dreams to life.

To Leanne and the amazing team at Octopus without whom this book would never have seen the light.